The Ultimate Gluten-Free Diet 2021

An Easy and Healthy Gluten FREE Cookbook

TABLE OF CONTENTS

CONCLUSION

CHAPTER 1: INTRODUCTION

WHAT IS GLUTEN, AND WHY IS IT BAD FOR YOU?

A healthy diet is the foundation of good health, which is why nutritious eating is so important for your body to feel good and to look good. Like a finely tuned racing car, your body needs just the right fuel (nutrition) and regular maintenance (a great lifestyle, positive mental attitude, favorable mental heath and regular exercise) to look impeccable and to achieve its maximum potential. If you put in the wrong fuel or lag behind on regular care and use, there is no way it can deliver its full muscle and performance, which is why nothing is more important than healthy eating!

Our organ systems rely on what we put inside our body to work in a manner that is most efficient, and if you don't take care of what you eat, then your body will deteriorate in health and won't function effectively. Not only will your body be affected, but your attitude and moods will also be greatly affected by how fit your body is. Someone who is not receiving proper nutrition or an adequate diet will tend to feel physically affected, experiencing lethargy, fatigue, and hence having an irritable and impatient disposition. Such disadvantages are damaging to well-being in the short term and the long-term, and individuals need to take immediate care of their health in order to live a happy, healthy life.

It doesn't matter whether you are a growing adolescent, a working parent or enjoying your retirement, healthy eating is the best present you can give to yourself and your body, and the extra effort is necessary to live a long and salubrious life. In our society, our eating habits have changed for the worst and our lifestyles have deteriorated. Junk foods have gained popularity, along with manufactured and packaged food that isn't as nutritious as we would like to believe.

Our busy lifestyles have caused us to have little time and little information and awareness about what food is good for us and what isn't, and the increased accessibility of convenience and processed foods has resulted in laziness, obesity, augmented health risks and a reduced lifespan. These negative affects have made our lives even more difficult because unhealthy eating has resulted in reduced energy and strength, dullness, a lack of attentiveness, and an increase in potential dangerous and damaging health problems. All this makes seeking proper nutrition even harder. It's a vicious cycle, and one which is difficult to get out of, but not impossible. With a little effort, we can free ourselves of this restrained and detrimental lifestyle and we can move into the arena of superior living with simple diets that can make our lives easier and healthier.

One of the foremost ways to begin on this road of healthy living is to consider the gluten-free lifestyle. Contrary to common misconceptions that a gluten-free living choice is expensive, restrictive, time consuming and hard to keep up with, it is one of the best diet options to contemplate and very easy with a little pre-planning and effort. Initially, such a diet may seem hard to implement, but as you read along in this book, you will discover an array of different types of gluten-free recipes, many of which are easy to make. They can even be upgraded to become main course meals with a bit of creativity and imagination. We will give you the information needed to make gluten-free living appealing, appetizing and very healthy.

Many grocery stores and restaurants have recently increased the availability of gluten-free options as compared to the number obtainable in the past, which makes keeping up with the diet relatively easy. This book will provide guidelines for shopping and eating out that will ensure that compliance with this diet is natural and comparatively effortless. Gluten-free living is a rapidly growing lifestyle change, surrounding which you will find a great deal of support which makes this diet possible to successfully execute and incorporate. This book will help you learn more about gluten-free living and help you make better choices about your diet.

As you read through this book, it is best to keep any predetermined concepts about food out of your mind, because any myths and false information about the benefits or uses of some food that you may have picked up previously will hinder the process of your understanding of the diet you think you need and the diet you actually need. Eliminate your previous knowledge of what constitutes "good food", and start afresh to frame your plan of action. We hope that our book helps you with the essential information, scientific facts, recipes and a course of action, and the encouragement that you need to go ahead with this decision. We are sure that as you read through our information, which has been carefully researched and compiled to suit your needs, you will find the necessary motivation and methods to not only welcome modifications in your routine but also to find the crucial means to do so.

For millions of people in the world, greater consciousness is leading to gluten-free diets compromising a daily part of their life. Today, we will show you why you should join this group of enlightened people. We will remove the barricades of misinformation and uncertainty to show you how to make this diet a viable possibility. If you have the motivation to embrace these changes, don't be afraid to do so! This book is here to guide you at every step to accomplish the greatest feat of healthy living. No matter what age or size you are, we will give you ways to adapt this diet to you specifically, and to your children and your friends so that everyone can enjoy the benefits of immaculate health. You can embark on this mission to live a great quality of life, but before you do so, it is important to explore what exactly gluten is, why it is harmful to your body, and what exactly a gluten-free lifestyle constitutes means.

CHAPTER 2: WHAT IS A GLUTEN-FREE LIFESTYLE?

If you ask people what exactly gluten is, most of them will be unable to explain. However, gluten is a significant part of the diet of an average person, and it is more common in the everyday food you eat than you may realize.

Gluten is a type of composite protein that is present in various foods including wheat, rye, barley and various cross breeds that are becoming increasingly popular. What makes gluten a problem for millions around the world is its presence in most of the staple and common foods of today, which is why problems related to gluten are so dangerous and hard to avoid. Almost all of our bread and baked goods, pizza, burgers, french fries, pastas, soups, sauces, cereals, and many vitamins, supplements and medications contain gluten, which makes it very difficult to avoid.

Millions of people all over the world experience problems in digesting gluten; suffering from undesirable reactions every time they attempt to consume it, such as heartburn, bloating, weakness and severe abdominal pain. For many, the adverse reaction to gluten consumption is much more severe, such that they are required to completely eliminate gluten from their diet, or otherwise undergo extremely deleterious reactions in their bodies, many of which could be fatal. Such intolerance to gluten is termed Celiac Disease.

Celiac disease is a severe autoimmune disease that affects every one in one hundred people in most parts of the world. Symptoms of Celiac Disease include chronic diarrhea, abdominal pain, weight loss, fatigue and lethargy, and joint pain, many of which result in difficulty in living a normal life. People suffering from Celiac Disease undergo a serious autoimmune responses when they expend too much gluten, causing damage to the intestines and leaving the patient unable to absorb any vitamins and essentials nutrients from the food, a condition that is often life-threatening. If Celiac Disease is left untreated, it advances to cause even more serious diseases and disorders such as infertility in women, osteoporosis, and bowel cancers. Since there is no cure for this disease, the best treatment that shows promise for a normal, safe life is a lifelong gluten-free diet. It is for the millions who experience difficulties in digesting gluten, and those who suffer from Celiac Disease, for whom this book is especially important.

If you have been facing any difficulties or digestion problems, it is recommended you see a doctor immediately. Despite the guidelines in this book, it is simply not enough to use these or the internet to self diagnose, especially in regards to a gluten problem, which is very serious and should not be taken lightly. The correct testing with a reliable doctor should be done since gluten-related diseases show symptoms that may be similar to other diseases and only a doctor can sufficiently point out what exact disease you may suffer with, if any at all.

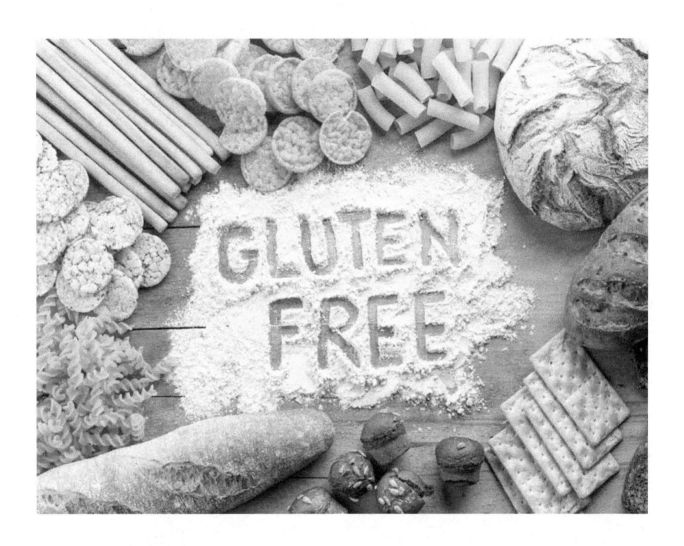

Figure 2.2: Symptoms of Celiac Disease

As you may have already realized, a gluten-free lifestyle is a way of living in which you completely exclude any foods containing gluten from your diet. The process of deciding which foods to eliminate is a little complex, but with research the problem can easily be overcome. For instance, oats don't have gluten in them, but due to the processing and packaging systems in our modern commercial markets, especially in certain states which require particular nutrients to be added to food which are lacking them, many packaged oats end up containing gluten. Hence going through labels and engaging in proper research is a very important constituent of a successful lifestyle plan.

However, it is important to conserve your appetite and make sure your stomach gets the taste and appeal it deserves regardless of following this diet. If you do not eat a wide variety of foods, then the plan is very hard to stick to and the body can become nutrient deficient or you can simply become tired, frustrated and exhausted with eating the same type of food over and over again. Hence it is important to eat a wide range of different types of dishes to ensure you don't feel constricted or limited to a few choices for meals, which is not healthy for any plan that you aim to stick to for the long term. Gluten-free dishes can be transformed into main courses, appetizers, side dishes and desserts that taste great and are still healthy. With the recipes included in this book, you can enjoy your food without feeling distaste or having to force yourself to eat any particular type of food.

With the plan this book will provide, you can have a proper gluten-free lifestyle that is not only easy to comply with, but also ensures a delicious diet that in the long term, will lead to a healthy and sustainable lifestyle which will not leave your body lacking the proper minerals, vitamins and fibers that are so very important for the daily functioning of the human body. Don't be alarmed, though! A large proportion of fresh fruits and vegetables, which are great antioxidants for removing toxins from the body and have abundant nutrients, are completely gluten-free. This means they will constitute a large amount of the plan, which only goes to show how this diet will give your life the healthy and nourishing turn that it needs. This diet plan will leave you satisfied and energetic, and healthier and fresher than you have ever been!

A word of caution: do not approach this diet with fear. A diet free of gluten might seem daunting, but there are many food choices out there that are great substitutes, and you won't have to give up a particular form of food completely. With the progress in today's day and age, even your favorite cakes and baked goods can be replicated using gluten-free alternatives, which goes to show how feasible a gluten-free diet is. Furthermore, it is a great idea to be visiting a doctor regularly while following this diet, because the diet has different effects on the bodies and metabolisms of different people. Some individuals might notice their symptoms disappear after switching to this diet, while others, owing to the severity of their condition, may notice prevalent symptoms even after removing gluten from their diet.

Many times, gluten-related diseases can damage the small intestine, which limits the advantages of gluten-free diets on the body. Hence, it is best to visit a doctor for dietary supplements to counteract the affect on the small intestine, which regulates the absorption of minerals and nutrients in the body and may result in malnourishment or weakness. Furthermore, any lack of nutrients should also be compensated for by visiting a physician or doctor to provide supplements for vitamins and minerals in the body, which can occur as a result of the body adjusting to the new gluten-free diet. As with any diet, care must be taken, but once it is smooth and running, the results are tremendous and worth the trouble.

CHAPTER 3: WHY IS A GLUTEN-FREE DIET GOOD FOR YOU AND YOUR BODY?

Individuals who suffer from gluten intolerance or diseases, like Celiac Disease that leaves the body literally unable to digest gluten, have to follow a gluten-free diet in order to live a normal and healthy life. Because of the way that their bodies react to any food substance containing gluten, it becomes a life necessity for their physical and mental well being to follow a diet that aims to completely eradicate gluten in their bodily systems.

Diseases such as Celiac Disease reject the processing of gluten in the body, and instead of recognizing it as a nutrient, it is recognized as a toxic substance, and so the body reacts in dangerous ways to remove it, many of which result in very serious health concerns. Even gluten allergies, though rare, are very hard to diagnose and hence in cases where allergic reactions are left unexplained, a gluten-free diet can be a good way to figure out if the allergic reaction is alleviated when the diet is being followed. Even though the harshness of the reaction of your body to gluten is relative to individual immune systems and gluten consumption, the reactions nonetheless need to be controlled. Excess gluten in the body also makes autism and migraines much worse.

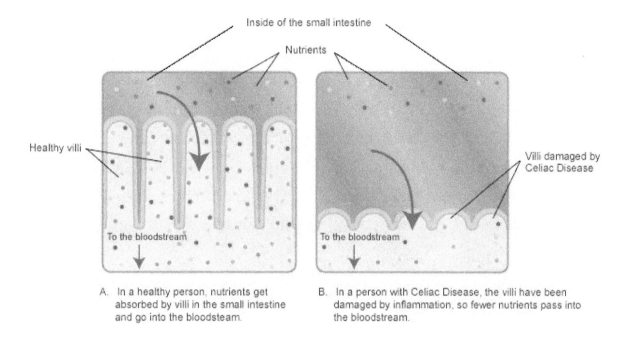

Figure 3.1: Damages on the intestines by untreated Celiac Disease

With the increasing awareness of gluten-related problems has come about a greater concern in the medical field, with professionals becoming more wary of gluten-related illnesses. Medical officers have begun to take special care to particularly test for the symptoms and presence of gluten reactions in the body. Recent years have shown a large amount of people, adults and children alike, who struggle with gluten-related problems, many of which have been left undiagnosed for years and have hence served as a nightmare and consistent barrier in normal living and good health in the lives of these individuals. It is recorded that 1 in 133 people suffer from one form or another of mild or severe Celiac Disease that has been left unidentified. Consumption of gluten damages the small intestine, leaving it unable to absorb nutrients that the body really requires.

One of the greatest dangers of Celiac Disease on your body comes from the fact that it is genetic and passed on within families, and also very hard to diagnose if not given proper knowledge, especially because in some people the symptoms present themselves as more visible manifestations in the form of some sort of physical affects, while in others the symptoms don't present themselves at all. Even though there are more than 300 possible symptoms of Celiac Disease and other gluten intolerant diseases, the most common, which should be kept constantly in mind are as follows:

- Chronic fatigue and a perpetual feeling of tiredness

- Depression and Anxiety

- Anemia and paleness of skin

- Stomach ache and severe bloating

- Weight fluctuations

- Diarrhea

- Infertility

- Pain in bones and muscles

- Abdominal pain

- Gassiness

- Headaches and nausea

In addition, children may suffer from other symptoms that become discernible at an early age, the most important being:

- Distended or painfully bloated abdomen

- Weight fluctuations or problems in gaining weight at their age group

- Short height; problems in attaining height for their age group

- Damaged teeth; dental enamel damage

- Behavioral changes

The advantage of a gluten-free diet is that it helps compensate for the damages incurred by consumption of gluten before the diagnosis of gluten digestive problems was given. It stops the continuing damage on the small intestine and over time can allow a person to make a full recovery. It puts the body and the digestive system on the right track to proper digestion, and gives time for the small intestine to heal from the damage it has incurred. The intestine will eventually resume its halted role of proper absorption of nutrients that will eventually allow the body to become healthier as it is now able to use all the nutrients that it consumes, unlike before.

Figure 3.2: Following Gluten-Free diet; Before and After

A gluten-free diet stops an exacerbation of health disorders that come about from continuing to eat gluten, such as malnutrition from inefficient absorption, neurological and mental problems, weakness in the bones and osteoporosis, and lymphoma and anemia. Furthermore, a gluten-free diet is the only cure for Celiac Disease. It is also the only known cure that reverses the damage caused by Dermatitis Herpetiformis, also called DH, which is a form of Celiac Disease that mainly affects the skin tissue. Medication helps little; it is only a drastic change in the sort of food the sufferer eats that causes the clearing up of skin and reversal of damage that has been caused.

However, a gluten-free lifestyle is not only exclusive to people who suffer from digestive disorders. Many people who do not suffer from such problems also voluntarily give up gluten. Some of these people are those who follow it as a preventative measure, owing to a family history of health problems related to gluten. Some merely opt for it to move to what they consider healthier sources, like natural fruits and vegetables, though for many, this may be temporary.

Even in cases where a gluten problem hasn't been diagnosed, and some problems such as mental or behavioral problems are unexplained, the gluten-free diet is a good way to move forward. Studies and surveys have shown that children who had some unexplained symptoms resembling those for gluten problems had massive health improvements after removing gluten from their diet. It helped them more than any medication or therapy, which goes to show the general health benefits of gluten removal from your diet. Furthermore, when such symptoms are left unexplained, it is a good idea to try a gluten-free diet and monitor any changes to figure out how beneficial it is, and eventually find the root cause of the issue based on whether the gluten-free diet has any effect on the child. Any improvements naturally mean continuing the diet and finding the proper cure for your child's health.

The benefits don't stop there! There are many studies that show that many other autoimmune diseases have symptoms that have been reduced by gluten-free diets. Such diseases include thyroid disease, multiple sclerosis and cystic fibrosis, and following gluten-free diets

have helped sufferers feel physically better and find that many of their symptoms have been massively reduced. These symptoms include severe body pains, fatigue, tiredness, anemia, breathing problems and many other issues that influence and hinder every aspect of a person's life. Following gluten-free diets massively help sufferers deal with the problems created by these symptoms, which is why this diet is so great to consider because of the impact it has on people who find no solace in any other medications or cures that more often than not, simply don't work out or help as much as they have promised.

Furthermore, the reason why starting a gluten-free lifestyle from an early age is good is because gluten-related diseases are very common and being ready for any sort of problems is always good. Plus parents with such diseases, which are genetic, should get their children used to such diets from an early age, as it is very likely that the children may also be sufferers of the disease when they grow up. Even before the onset of the disease, minor problems like bloating and gas that often cause discomfort can be relieved with the gluten-free diet that simply makes the children feel better physically, since these problems cause discomfort and make it hard to concentrate on social interactions and your work. Getting rid of these problems makes a person feel much more fresh and in a better mood.

Gluten-free diets are also the supreme winners when it comes to weight loss. The biggest problem in shedding pounds is the constant urge to eat sweets and the craving for sweet stuff. However, gluten-free diets include a lot of fresh fruits, which reduce cravings for more fatty, sweet stuff, and reduce appetite as a whole if the diet is changed and

molded to become a weight loss plan. Also, because this diet is very natural and long term, the weight lost is often lost for good since the main causes of weight gain, such as empty calories or other snacks and processed foods, are eliminated in a gluten-free diet. These changes are exactly what are needed to lose weight while simultaneously feeling nourished and fresh.

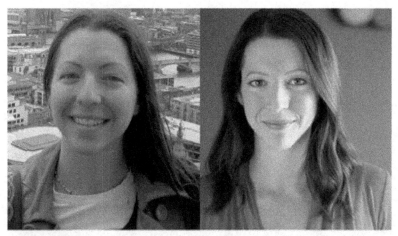

Pre-Gluten-Free ('07) & Gluten-Free (11/15/13)

Figure 3.3: Gluten-Free Diet; Before and After

Additionally, most people have reported that gluten-free plans are easier to stick to than other diets which are too harsh and many of which are simply fad diets. Gluten-free diets, these people have reported, give a feeling of fullness and freshness and also help people lose weight. The reasons behind why the diet is so successful for keeping your body fit and rid of extra fat are very simple. Over a longer period of time, cravings go away due to the habit of eating fresh fruit and other fulfilling foods, all of which allows for healthy food choices.

Gluten-free diets are also diets that remove most processed food from our daily lives, which means there are fewer unnecessary carbs

and less sugar intake that the body will eventually store as fat. Gluten-free diets also provide a lot of energy and freshness, which gives people the power and motivation they need to begin exercising. Laziness may have prevented them before, but this diet will give them the power to reach their goals. Eventually, we can conclude that with a gluten-free diet, better health means improved moods and mental health, all of which leads to a happier and physically fitter person. Medical experts haven't given this diet in-depth research and analysis, which is why there is very little media attention, however, studies have shown many success stories highlighting how gluten-free diets were the only diets for some people that let them lose weight, which shows the efficiency of this diet and why it is so great for the body.

Gluten-free diets aren't as hard or time consuming as popular opinion might state. They're easy to make once you understand what you should eat and what you shouldn't. It also doesn't mean large expenditure on food as gluten-free food is not expensive to buy, and with the trend of more and more gluten-free food available in restaurants, eating out has also become easier. For people who travel a lot, a little research can make life very easy. You can use the Internet to discover gluten-free foods in the area, and restaurants and food choices available that fit your diet. A little work can go a long way, and once you know which places to eat at and what to eat and what to avoid, even travelling will not serve as a barrier to your diet.

Given all these benefits, it's advisable for all parents to pass on this knowledge to their children. At an early age, children should learn to

make good food choices, and parents should encourage them. You should guide your children about the nutritional values of several common foods and make sure they know how to check labels and decipher which foods are healthy to eat and which are not. Make sure they don't hesitate to ask an adult when confused about their food choices! Also make sure that visiting friends or going out to parties does not stop your children from abandoning these diets. Even though it may sound hectic, the long-term benefits are worth it. For example, you can make special arrangements for children when they go to places where gluten-free stuff may not be available, such as sending homemade food. Sometimes when kids suffer from a serious gluten-related disease, then this becomes a necessity, but in other cases it is still very important to make sure they comply with the diet because once they go off track, it is very easy to lose sight of the importance of the diet and abandon it.

We should also make sure that older individuals in and over their 60s are taken care of. If they require gluten-free diets, we should make sure that they are given those diets promptly and always, even if they are in someone else's care or in an old age or assisted care facility. This is important because diseases in the elderly are even more dangerous due to their old age and weaker immune system, and hence can become extremely serious which is why prevention and cure needs to be taken very seriously.

However, the diet needs to be complemented by exercise for its maximum potential to be revealed. Daily exercise is important for individuals no matter what their age. Gluten-free diets are great, but

exercise still needs to be part of the daily routine so that all the extra energy you gain can be put to good use, and generally exercise is crucial for a good body, and sustaining a healthy weight. A diet's success can only be measured when exercise is included, because physical exercise is a must. Many people feel lethargic when they don't work out often, so when you shift to a gluten-free diet, put that added vitality to good use by engaging in physical stimulation. Yet again, don't forget to refer to your doctor because his expertise may be needed in figuring out how a blanket policy can be molded to suit individual cases.

Make these changes to your life slowly and gradually; changes that are too fast are often harder to stick with. Slow changes help you ease into a new lifestyle and are hence the more preferred way forward. Pay great attention to your eating habits and slowly let them change. After you have settled into your diet, ease into the habit of exercising until it becomes a part of your routine that you don't necessarily have to force upon yourself. Once the diet and exercise become an integrated part of your life, it will be easy to continue with that lifestyle with long lasting, excellent results.

CHAPTER 4: WHAT TO EAT AND WHAT NOT TO EAT

Before we begin discussing what foods are off limits for your diet plan, it's worth mentioning that gluten is not only present in the foods that you ingest, but also in many household items, which may be equally harmful for your body. This is why care needs to be taken in looking into what sort of products you use, whether gluten has been included in their manufacture, and hence whether they need to be remove from daily use. Some common household items should be checked before they can be used again, however every item should be evaluated by checking its label for the composition of the product. Such common items include:

- Glue or any sort of adhesive

- Lip balms or chapsticks

- Toothpaste, mouth fresheners and mouth washes

- Any and all sorts of medicines, such as herbal medicines, prescriptions and over the counter

- Bubble gum and may types of candy

What this section primarily serves to do is to give guidelines as to how to shop for gluten-free products and how to make sure that when you are eating out at restaurants, you order food that does not compromise the lifestyle that you have chosen for yourself.

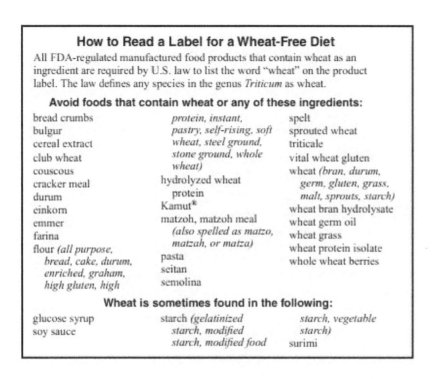

How to Read a Label for a Wheat-Free Diet

All FDA-regulated manufactured food products that contain wheat as an ingredient are required by U.S. law to list the word "wheat" on the product label. The law defines any species in the genus *Triticum* as wheat.

Avoid foods that contain wheat or any of these ingredients:

bread crumbs
bulgur
cereal extract
club wheat
couscous
cracker meal
durum
einkorn
emmer
farina
flour *(all purpose,
    bread, cake, durum,
    enriched, graham,
    high gluten, high*

*protein, instant,
    pastry, self-rising, soft
    wheat, steel ground,
    stone ground, whole
    wheat)*
hydrolyzed wheat
    protein
Kamut®
matzoh, matzoh meal
    *(also spelled as matzo,
    matzah, or matza)*
pasta
seitan
semolina

spelt
sprouted wheat
triticale
vital wheat gluten
wheat *(bran, durum,
    germ, gluten, grass,
    malt, sprouts, starch)*
wheat bran hydrolysate
wheat germ oil
wheat grass
wheat protein isolate
whole wheat berries

Wheat is sometimes found in the following:

glucose syrup
soy sauce

starch *(gelatinized
    starch, modified
    starch, modified food*

*starch, vegetable
    starch)*
surimi

Figure 4.1: Guide to Gluten-Free Foods

First and foremost, know that planning is the key to a successful diet. Planning means you are always prepared for your meals and will never be catapulted into a situation where a lack of time forces you to make an unhealthy choice. Plan every meal and every snack so that you can track what sort of food you are eating and when. Buy all your products before-hand. This has become easier, because more stores have started to offer gluten-free products than before, and the variety of products in the market is steadily increasing. Studies show that availability and variety will continue to increase in the coming years. Especially with online shopping, finding items you require has become easier, or you can simply order or ask for more stock as more stores provide that choice to their customers.

The first step is to know which foods you can eat. This might feel odd to you as most guidelines start off with identifying which food is off limits. However, people who need to begin long-term gluten-free lifestyles begin with knowing what food they can eat, and not what food they are giving up, because starting off with that might make the whole process seem unnecessarily daunting.

The first thing you should do when you enter a store is to read labels carefully! Different brands of the same products may contain gluten, so you need to check labels and see which ones are gluten-free products and hence suitable for your diet. It is important to understand that there is a difference between gluten-free products and low gluten products; your diet needs to exclude low gluten products as well.

Buy as many fruits and vegetables as you want, they are foods that should definitely always be on your "to eat" list, because they are not processed and are all gluten-free. All green vegetables and fresh fruits, as well as sweet and white potatoes, and peas and dry beans, are acceptable and great choices to consider as part of your daily diet.

Most dairy products are also free of gluten and hence great choices. Milk, cheese and plain yoghurt are free of gluten, except some processed types, so you need to take care before you buy by asking and evaluating labels. For example, some flavored yoghurt may contain gluten, so checking labels is important, and blue cheese and some other processed cheese products may also have wheat in them, which is why they can't be consumed, hence take care to check all processed foods for the ingredients used in their manufacture.

Meat, fish, pork and poultry can also become a part of your diet as long as you are selective. Buy only lean cuts of meat, pork and poultry, and buy fresh fish and seafood. Canned and frozen products of any of the aforementioned foods are processed and will likely contain gluten; some may not, but it is mostly dependent on individual companies and hence labels always need to be referred to. The best option would be to always buy fresh products as they are gluten-free and generally more healthy and retain more nutrients than those which are no longer fresh and have been frozen, canned or processed in any other way.

The hardest task perhaps in shopping is finding gluten-free grains, as a lot of common grains contain gluten. Research and asking around grocery shops will lead you to discover and select grains that are gluten-free, and you can then choose between what varieties of the grains you want to eat. Sometimes, common grains that usually contain gluten do not due to different processing methods, and hence you will find that different types of processed grain such as wild, brown and white rice may not contain gluten. This leaves consumers with a lot of choice and, even though they are limited by a diet, their food choices continue to remain vast and many.

When you're dining out, a different type of care is required in choosing adequate foods. Research in this aspect is important to find

out which restaurants in your area offer gluten-free dishes, or may make such dishes upon request. The same goes for when you are travelling. Planning beforehand means you can dine out without compromising your diet. However, there are some common dishes that are gluten-free anyway, so you can still order without specifying the need for it to be free of gluten. Dishes such as salads, seafood dishes, dishes with meat with a side of vegetables, and baked potato dishes are common items that are also gluten-free. You should ask what sort of oil they are cooked in as some oils contain gluten, but that shouldn't be an issue as most places use gluten-free oils or have gluten-free oils that can be used instead.

What you need to be especially careful about in restaurants is avoiding dishes with exotic sauces and marinades. Almost all sauces have large amounts of gluten in them and it is best to simply avoid dishes that give you ample sauces. Saucy foods mean more gluten means when you go home from the restaurant that day, you will not get a good night's sleep due to the body disturbance it will cause. You can choose to be extra careful with sauces, or you can ask for dishes and eliminate the sauces. Both are good ways to ensure gluten-full sauces are excluded from your diet.

However, you should most probably leave out baked wheat or bread goods and crackers, since they have large amounts of gluten and almost no present alternatives. This also goes for beer; it contains huge amounts of gluten from the grains that are used to make it, hence beer needs to be positively off limits. What you can instead go for is champagne and wine. Furthermore, various places offer gluten-free drinks and upon research, you can discover some common mixed drinks that do not contain gluten.

The best part is that a gluten-free diet will not mean you have to give up dessert. In fact, even with this specific diet, there are some tasty choices for dessert that will quench your cravings for sweets. You can ask for a menu of gluten-free desserts from restaurants. If not, there are common foods like flourless cakes that you can eat instead. Sorbet, ice cream, fresh fruit and sherbet are very common and tasty alternatives for dessert, which will almost always be available at grocery stores or wherever you are dining out.

Other common practices you should adopt include the saying: better safe than sorry. Some labels may be ambiguous about containing gluten and it is best to be cautious and not buy them, as compared to suffering a reaction after eating them. You can always research that product later and then choose whether to buy it or not. Slowly and steadily, as you become aware of what you should eat and what you shouldn't, it will become second nature for you to easily find gluten-free products on your shopping trips and whenever you eat out.

There are a few products that you should keep stocked at home, as they are usually needed for gluten-free recipes. These include:

- Brown or white rice

- Xantham gum

- Guar gum

- Quinoa

- Gluten-free crackers

- Gluten-free snacks

- Gluten-free flour

- Gluten-free baking mix

- Gluten-free bread crumbs

Most of these products can be used to replace other gluten products in dishes. Here are some ways to go about using these products in different ways to replace common gluten parts of recipes:

- For thickening, use gluten-free baking mix

- For binding, use xantham or guar gum

- For breading, use gluten-free bread crumbs or crushed potato chips

- Gluten-free baking mix can be used as a replacement for flour

CHAPTER 5: HOW TO KEEP A GLUTEN-FREE DIET ON BUDGET

There are several very simple tips that are helpful when keeping to a gluten-free diet on a budget. It is important, like every other activity involving money, that you should budget your diet, as at some points you may feel that it may get expensive.

One way to budget is to make sure that when you buy several products that expire early or are perishable, you should use them immediately, otherwise they will waste away, along with the money you spent on them. Secondly, if any one member of the family is on a gluten-free diet, don't spend extra money trying to make separate food for that person and the rest of the family. Due to genetics, if you suffer from gluten intolerance, your children may as well, so it will generally be a better idea to have your whole family follow the same diet. Even if that is not the case, try to make dishes that are agreeable to the whole family but need only small alterations for the individual for whom the dish should be gluten-free. This saves money as the whole family will eat the same type of food and extra money does not need to be spent catering for that one person.

Try to buy foods in bulk or on sale as this always saves money. Properly store whatever materials you buy in bulk so that they can be used for longer without being spoilt and that money is saved, not only on directly buying the product but also on saving money that will be spent on fuel and time that will be wasted on grocery trips. Mostly however, maintaining a gluten-free diet is only as expensive as a normal diet so there should not be too many problems with budgeting.

One online resource we recommend you to look at is this:

http://www.celiaccentral.org/celiac-disease-in-the-news/gluten-free-menu-planning-on-a-budget-new-printable-guide-released-9849/

This online resource leads to a printable guide covering Gluten-free Menu Planning on a budget. It helps readers understand the essentials of how to plan their diet in an organized and sustainable way, as well as giving sample diet plans to supplement their knowledge.

Online shopping should also be an important part of your budgeting. Online shopping is very easy, and all you have to do is find the right website. Once you have found a website that delivers where you live, all you need to do is type in what you need, add it to your cart, and buy it. The benefit of online shopping is that you can easily use multiple websites to find different varieties of foods from different companies and compare prices and quantities. This comparing is easy instead of walking to different stores to find different types of the same food. Online shopping helps compare prices and prepare an accurate shopping list of the best deals you can find and buy, and have them delivered to your house without you yourself having to make any extra trouble. Anyone wanting to budget their gluten-free lifestyle should seriously consider online shopping as a crucial part of managing their diet.

One of the best ways to budget your gluten-free diet is to consider planning ahead and making a list of gluten-free products you need. Tally the products and their prices with the budget you have, and slowly weed out unnecessary products till you have a list which matches the amount of money you can expend on gluten-free food. Use this same budget or as a budget that suits your need for the rest of the months too, adding and subtracting foods from your list depending on their price, and your preference.

One way you can do this is using a budget calculator. One good budget calculator that may be used online can be accessed through the following link.

https://www.eatthismuch.com/

CHAPTER 6: GLUTEN-FREE RECIPES FOR BREAKFAST

Delicious Gluten-Free Pancakes (Makes 5 pancakes)

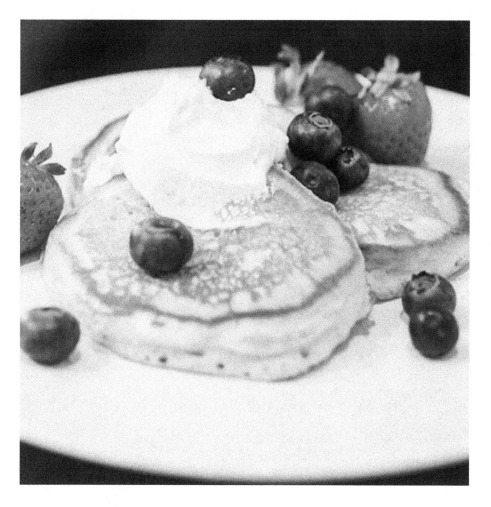

Ingredients:

- ½ cup rice flour

- 1 and a ½ tablespoons tapioca flour

- ½ packet sugar substitute

- 1/6 cup potato starch

- 2 tablespoons dry buttermilk powder

- ¾ teaspoons baking powder

- ¼ teaspoon salt

- ¼ teaspoon baking soda

- ¼ teaspoon xanthan gum

- 1 egg

- 1 cup water

- 1 and a ½ tablespoons canola oil

  <u>Preparation time:</u> 20 minutes

  <u>Cooking time:</u> 15 minutes

  <u>Total time:</u> 35 minutes

  <u>Method:</u>

- In a large bowl, sift together the rice flour, potato starch, tapioca flour, dry buttermilk powder, sugar substitute, baking soda, baking powder, xanthan gum, and salt.

- Mix in the eggs, water and oil till the mixture is smooth and well mixed. No lumps/few lumps should remain.

- Heat a large non-stick pan or well oiled skillet over medium to high heat. Pour 4 tablespoons batter into the pan and cook until bubbles form on the surface. Flip and cook both sides till crispy and golden brown.

- Do the same till all batter is used. Serve with sides of your choice, such as fresh fruit, jam, etc., or top with honey, blueberries, and chopped almonds.

Ham and Cheese Breakfast Quiche (makes 5 servings)

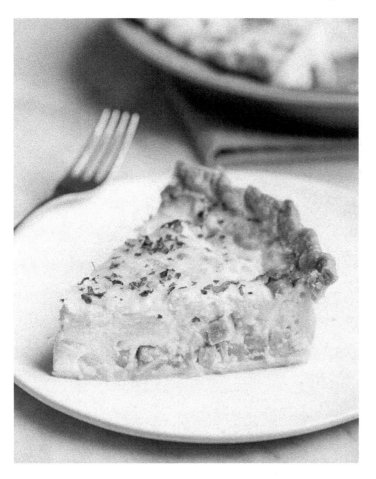

Ingredients:

- 2 packages or 12 ounces of frozen hash brown potatoes

- ½ cup heavy whipping cream

- 2 eggs

- 1 cup cooked diced ham

- 1/3 cup melted butter

- 1 cup shredded Monterey Jack cheese

Preparation time: 20 minutes

Cooking time: 55 minutes

Total time: 1 hour and 15 minutes

Method:

- Preheat the oven to 425 degrees Fahrenheit, or 220 degrees Celsius.

- Press the potatoes to squeeze out any excess liquid or moisture and add to a small bowl. Combine them with melted butter or margarine. Mix well.

- Line the bottom and sides of an ungreased 10-inch pie pan or baking dish with this mixture.

- Bake for 25 minutes in the preheated oven.

- Remove the baking dish from the oven and arrange the cheese and ham over the potatoes uniformly.

- In another bowl, beat the eggs and cream until smooth and fluffy, and pour over the ham and cheese in the baking dish.

- Return the dish to the oven and bake for 30 minutes, till the custard has completely set and browned slightly.

Corned Beef Hash (for 12 servings)

ngredients:

- 12 large potatoes, peeled and diced

- 2 cups of beef broth

- 2 cans or 24 ounces of corned beef, cut up into chunks

- 2 medium to large onions, chopped

  Preparation time: 10 minutes

  Cooking time: 30 minutes

  Total time: 40 minutes

  Method:

- In a large and deep pan or iron skillet, combine the potatoes, beef broth, onions and corned beef over medium heat. Cover the pan and simmer the mixture until the potatoes are soft and of mashing consistency, and the liquid has almost completely evaporated. Mix the contents well and serve hot.Feta Eggs (for 8 servings)

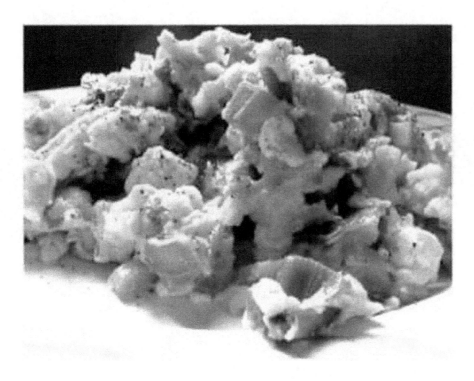

Ingredients:

- 8 eggs, beaten

- ½ cup chopped tomatoes

- 4 tablespoons crumbled feta cheese

- 2 tablespoons butter

- Salt and pepper to taste

Preparation time: 10 minutes

Cooking time: 5 minutes

Total time: 15 minutes

Method:

- Melt the butter in a large pan or an iron skillet over medium heat and add onions. Sauté the onions till they are translucent.

- Pour the beaten eggs into the skillet and cook well, stirring constantly with a spoon in order to scramble the eggs.

- When the eggs appear cooked, and are light, fluffy and brownish, stir in the feta cheese and chopped tomatoes. Season with salt and pepper to taste. Cook until the cheese has melted, and serve hot, with bread of your choice.

American Frittata (for 8 servings)

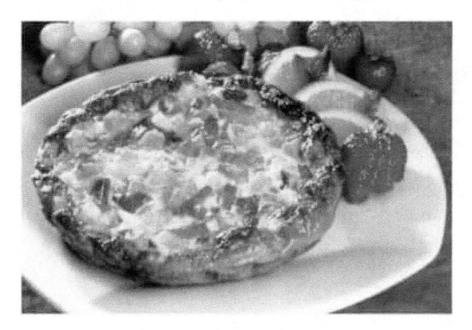

Ingredients:

* 8 eggs, beaten

* ¾ cup Cheddar cheese, shredded

* ¾ cup cubed ham

* 1 small onion, sliced

* 4 potatoes, peeled and cubed

* 1 tablespoon of vegetable oil

* Salt and pepper to taste

Preparation time: 15 minutes

Cooking time: 15 minutes

<u>Total time:</u> 30 minutes

<u>Method:</u>

- In a saucepan, add salt and water and boil. Add the potatoes to the boiling water and cook till they are tender and soft but still firm, which will be about 5 minutes. Drain the water and set the potatoes aside to cool.

- Preheat the oven to 350 degrees Fahrenheit or 175 degrees Celsius.

- In a large pan or an iron skillet, add oil and heat over medium heat. Add the onions and cook slowly stirring occasionally, until the onions are soft and translucent.

- To the onions, add the eggs, ham, drained potatoes, salt and pepper, and mix. Cook over medium heat until the eggs are firm on the bottom, which will be about 5 minutes.

- After the mixture has cooked, top the frittata with shredded cheese and bake in the preheated oven for 10 minutes, or till the cheese has fully melted and the eggs are firm.

Zucchini and Eggs (for 4 servings)

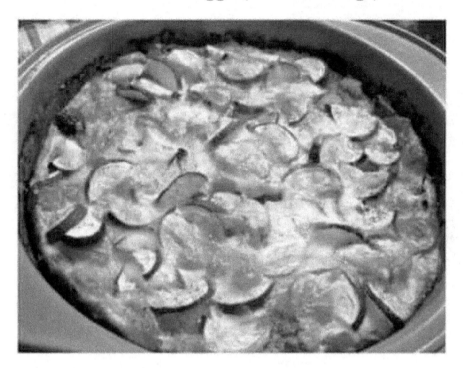

Ingredients:

- 4 zucchinis, sliced

- 8 teaspoons of olive oil

- 4 beaten eggs

- Salt and pepper to taste

Preparation time: 5 minutes

Cooking time: 5 minutes

Total time: 10 minutes

<u>Method:</u>

- Heat a pan or an iron skillet over medium heat. Add the oil and when the oil is hot, add the zucchinis and sauté until they are tender.

- In the skillet, spread out the zucchinis in an even layer, and pour the beaten egg evenly on top. Cook on medium heat until the eggs are fluffy and firm. Season with salt and pepper to taste. Serve hot or warm and with bread of your choice.

Gluten-free Waffles (for 10 servings)

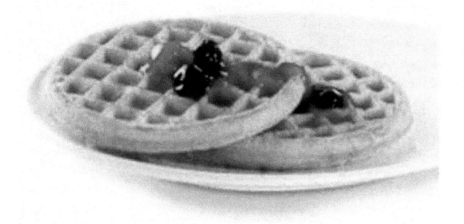

Ingredients:

- 3 cups of sorghum flour

- 2 chicken eggs, yolk and white separated

- 2 duck eggs, yolk and white separated

- 1 cup of tapioca starch

- 2 teaspoons xanthan gum

- 4 teaspoons of baking powder

- ¼ cups of white sugar

- ½ teaspoon of salt

- 2 teaspoons of vanilla extract

- ½ cup unsweetened applesauce

- 3 and ½ cups of unsweetened vanilla flavored almond milk

  Preparation time: 15 minutes

  Cooking time: 15 minutes

  Total time: 30 minutes

  Method:

- Preheat a waffle iron pan and grease with butter, oil, or cooking spray.

- In a bowl, mix together the sorghum flour, baking powder, white sugar, tapioca starch, xanthan gum and salt.

- Beat the whites of the duck and chicken eggs using an electric mixer or beater, until they are white and foamy, and stiff and soft peaks form. Do this by lifting the beater or whisk you are using straight up, and the egg whites should form soft stiff peaks rather than sharp peaks.

- Beat the duck and chicken egg yolks, vanilla extract, applesauce and almond milk in a bowl. Continue beating while simultaneously adding the flour mixture, and blend until no lumps are left and the mixture is smooth.

- Using a spatula or metal spoon, fold the egg whites into the batter.

- Pour 2/3 cups of the batter onto the waffle iron, and cook until golden brown. Repeat till mixture is all used up. Serve hot.

Sarah's Applesauce (for 8 servings)

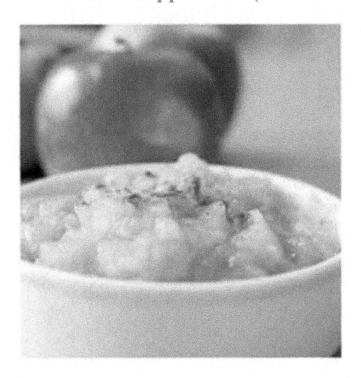

Ingredients:

- 8 apples, all peeled, cored and diced

- 1 and a ½ cups of water

- ½ cup of white sugar

- 1 teaspoon of ground cinnamon

Preparation time: 10 minutes

Cooking time: 20 minutes

Total time: 30 minutes

Method:

- Combine the chopped apples, water, sugar and cinnamon in a saucepan over medium heat.

- Cook for 15 to 20 minutes until the apples are soft. Check with a fork.

- Allow the mixture to cool. When cool, mash the lumps of apple in the mixture with a fork or potato masher. Serve hot or cool with bread of your choice.

Breakfast Sausage (for 12 servings)

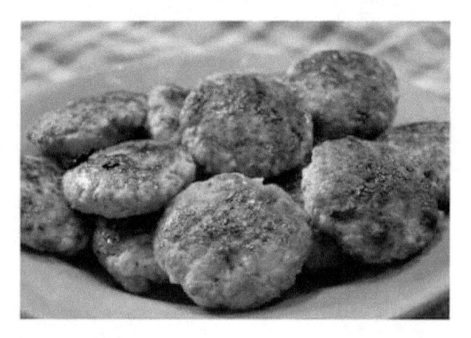

Ingredients:

- 2 tablespoons of brown sugar

- 4 teaspoons of dried sage

- 4 teaspoons of salt

- ½ teaspoon of dried marjoram

- 4 pounds ground pork

- ¼ teaspoons crushed red pepper flakes

- 2 pinches ground cloves

- 2 teaspoons ground black pepper

Preparation time: 10 minutes

Cooking time: 15 minutes

Total time: 25 minutes

<u>Method:</u>

- Combine the marjoram, brown sugar, sage, salt, ground black pepper, crushed red pepper and cloves in a small bowl, and mix well.

- Add the mixed spices to the pork in a large bowl and mix well with your hands. Combine into a mixture that can be molded. Use your hands to form round flat patties.

- Grease a large iron skillet or non-stick pan with butter or oil, and sauté the patties over medium to high heat for 5 minutes per side. Use a meat thermometer to cook the patties till the internal pork temperature reaches 160 degrees Fahrenheit or 173 degrees Celsius, and when the outside of the patties are crisp and brown.

Baby Spinach Omelet (for 2 servings)

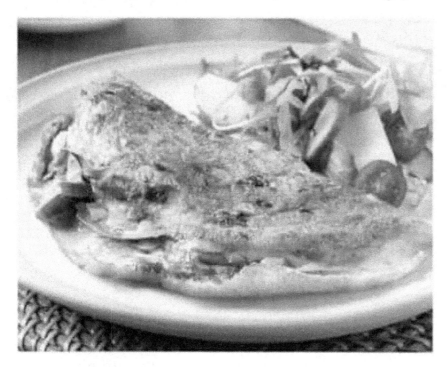

Ingredients:

- 4 eggs

- ¼ teaspoons of ground nutmeg

- ½ teaspoon of onion powder

- 2 cups of torn baby spinach leaves

- 2 tablespoons of grated Parmesan cheese

- Salt and Pepper to taste

Preparation time: 6 minutes

Cooking time: 9 minutes

Total time: 15 minutes

Method:

- Using a fork or beater, beat the eggs well in a bowl. Stir in the baby spinach leaves and grated Parmesan cheese. Season the eggs with salt and pepper, along with onion powder, and nutmeg.

- Grease an iron skillet or non stick pan with cooking spray, oil or butter, and over medium to high heat, cook the egg mixture about 3 minutes on each side, until the egg is set. After both sides have browned, reduce the heat to low and cook an additional 2 to 3 minutes per side to ensure the egg is cooked well inside out. Serve hot or warm with bread of your choice.

CHAPTER 7: GLUTEN-FREE RECIPES FOR LUNCH AND DINNER

JUICY ROASTED CHICKEN (FOR 6 SERVINGS)

CABBAGE ROLL CASSEROLE (FOR 6 SERVINGS)

LAMB CHOPS WITH BALSAMIC REDUCTION (FOR 8 SERVINGS)

GRILLED MARINATED SHRIMP (FOR 12 SERVINGS)

SIRLOIN STEAK WITH GARLIC BUTTER (FOR 8 SERVINGS)

CHILI-LIME CHICKEN KABOBS (FOR 8 SERVINGS)

FISH FILLETS ITALIANO (FOR 8 SERVINGS)

CHICKPEA CURRY (FOR 8 SERVINGS)

BEEF POT ROAST (FOR 8 SERVINGS)

PORCUPINES (FOR 10 SERVINGS)

GRILLED ROCK LOBSTER TAILS (FOR 8 SERVINGS)

LENTILS AND SPINACH (FOR 8 SERVINGS)

MUSHROOM RISOTTO (FOR 8 SERVINGS)

SCOTT URE'S CLAMS AND GARLIC (FOR 4 SERVINGS)

ROSEMARY BRAISED LAMB SHANKS (FOR 4 SERVINGS)

GRILLED SEA BASS (FOR 12 SERVINGS)

HARVEST RICE DISH (FOR 6 SERVINGS)

QUICK CHICKEN AND WINE (FOR 6 SERVINGS)

BAKED TILAPIA IN GARLIC AND OLIVE OIL (FOR 8 SERVINGS)

MAPLE GLAZED RIBS (FOR 6 SERVINGS)

Juicy Roasted Chicken (for 6 servings)

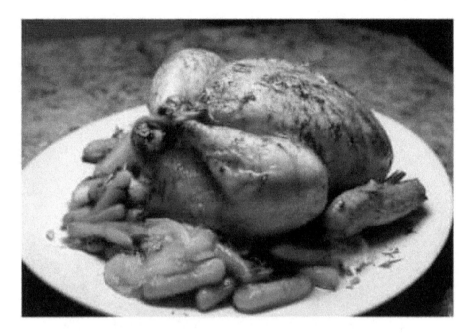

Ingredients:

- 1 whole chicken or 3 pound chicken, innards removed

- 1 stalk of celery with leaves removed

- ½ cup margarine, cut into small blocks

- 1 tablespoon onion powder

- Salt and pepper to taste

Preparation time: 10minutes

Cooking time: 1 hour and 15 minutes

Total time: 1 hour and 40 minutes

Method:

- Preheat oven to 350 degrees Fahrenheit or 175 degrees Celsius.

- Grease a roasting pan with butter, cooking spray or oil. Place chicken in the roasting pan, and season inside and outside with salt and pepper.

- Sprinkle onion powder inside and over the chicken. Rub 3 tablespoons margarine inside the chicken cavity. Arrange blocks of the remaining margarine around the chicken's exterior.

- Cut the celery into 4 – 5 pieces and place inside the chicken cavity.

- Bake in the preheated oven for 1 hour and 15 minutes. Use a meat thermometer to ensure a minimum internal temperature of 180 degrees Fahrenheit or 82 degrees Celsius.

- Remove the chicken from the oven and baste with melted margarine and the drippings from the roasting pan. Cover the pan and chicken with aluminum foil, and allow it to sit for 30 minutes before serving. Roasted chicken can be served with mashed potatoes or a side of boiled vegetables or boiled rice.

Cabbage Roll Casserole (for 6 servings)

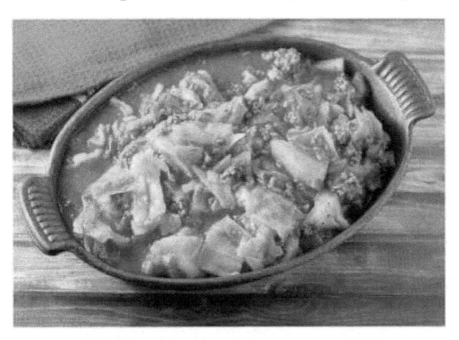

Ingredients:

- 1 pound of ground beef

- ½ cup of chopped onions

- 14 ounces of ½ can of tomato sauce

- ½ cup uncooked white rice (or any gluten-free rice of your choice)

- 1 can or 7 ounces of beef broth

- 1 and ¾ pounds of chopped cabbage

- ½ teaspoon salt

Preparation time: 10 minutes

Cooking time: 1 hour and 30 minutes

Total time: 1 hour and 40 minutes

<u>Method:</u>

- Preheat an oven to 350 degrees Fahrenheit or 175 degrees Celsius.

- In a large non-stick pan or greased skillet, add oil and ground beef, and cook over medium to high heat till the meat is browned. Drain the fat from the pan.

- Combine the onion, salt, rice, cabbage, and tomato sauce in a large mixing bowl. Add the meat and mix well. Pour the mixture into a baking dish.

- Pour the broth over the meat mixture, cover the dish, and bake in the preheated oven for 1 hour. Remove the dish, stir the contents, and bake for another 30 minutes. Serve hot.

Lamb Chops with Balsamic Reduction (for 8 servings)

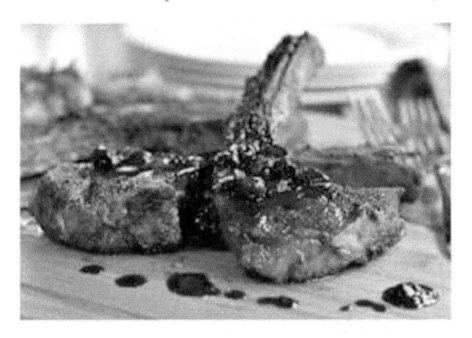

Ingredients:

- 8 lamb chops, each ¾ inches thick

- 2/3 cup of aged balsamic vinegar

- 1 and a ½ cups chicken broth

- ½ cup of minced shallots

- 2 tablespoons of butter

- 2 tablespoons of olive oil

- 1 and a ½ teaspoons dried rosemary

- ½ teaspoon of dried basil

- 1 teaspoon dried thyme

- Salt and Pepper to taste

  <u>Preparation Time:</u> 10 minutes + 15 minutes

  <u>Cooking Time:</u> 15 minutes

  <u>Total time:</u> 40 minutes

  <u>Method:</u>

- Mix the rosemary, thyme, basil, salt and pepper in a small bowl, and rub this mixture onto the lamb chops evenly and generously on both sides. Put the lamb chops on a plate, cover them with a plastic or metallic cover, and set aside for 15 minutes to allow the chops to absorb the flavor from the spices.

- In a large skillet, heat olive oil over medium to high heat and cook the lamb chops for 3 to 4 minutes each side for medium rare meat, or as preferred. Put the chops on a serving platter and keep warm.

- In the same skillet, brown the shallots. Add the vinegar and stir in the chicken broth while grating off the lamb bits from the surface of the pan using a wooden spoon. Cook for 4 to 5 minutes on medium to high heat, until the sauce has thickened and condensed by half. Remove from the heat and stir in the butter. Pour the sauce over the lamb chops, and serve hot. Garnish with mint.

Grilled Marinated Shrimp (for 12 servings)

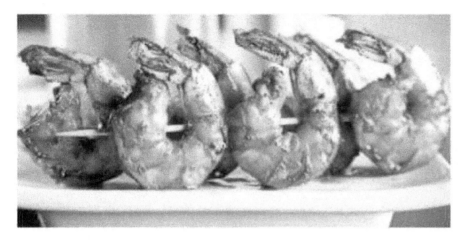

Ingredients:

- 2 cups of olive oil

- 4 pounds of large shrimp, peeled and deveined with the tails attached

- ½ cup of fresh parsley, chopped

- 6 cloves of garlic, minced

- 2 tablespoons of tomato paste

- 4 teaspoons of dried oregano

- 4 tablespoons of hot pepper sauce

- Freshly squeezed lemon juice from 2 lemons

- 2 teaspoons of ground black pepper

- 2 teaspoons of salt

  Preparation Time: 30 minutes + 2 hours

  Cooking Time: 10 minutes

<u>Total time:</u> 2 hours and 40 minutes

<u>Method:</u>

- Mix the olive oil, lemon juice, hot sauce, tomato paste, parsley, garlic, oregano, salt and black pepper in a bowl. Remove ¼ cup of the mixture for basting. Pour the remaining mixture into an airtight plastic bag with the shrimp and seal it. Refrigerate for 2 hours.

- Grease the grill with butter, oil or cooking spray and preheat the grill on medium to low heat. Shake the plastic bag well so the marinade covers the shrimp. Remove the shrimp from the bag. Using wooden skewers, pierce the shrimp, first from the tail and out from the head. Skewer all the shrimp.

- Cook the shrimp on each side for 5 minutes till they become opaque, basting occasionally with the saved marinade. Cook till well done, and serve hot, on a plate of pasta or egg fried rice.

Sirloin Steak with Garlic Butter (for 8 servings)

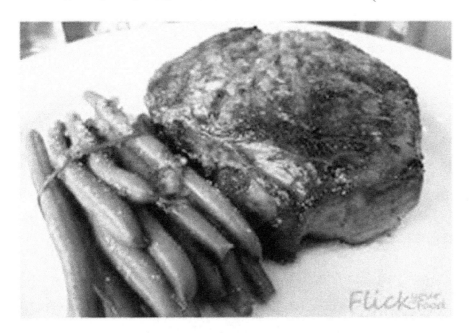

Ingredients:

- 4 pounds beef top sirloin steaks

- 2 teaspoons of garlic powder

- ½ cup of butter

- 4 cloves of garlic, minced

- Salt and pepper to taste

Preparation Time: 20 minutes

Cooking Time: 10 minutes

Total time: 30 minutes

<u>Method:</u>

- Grease a grill with butter or oil, or preheat an outdoor grill on medium to high heat.

- Melt butter in a small saucepan over medium to low heat, and add the garlic powder and minced garlic. Stir well.

- Rub salt and pepper on each side of the steak. Cook the steak on the grill for 4 to 5 minutes per side, till brown, or to your preferred doneness. Once cooked, transfer to serving plates. Top the steaks with the garlic and butter mixture, and garnish with chopped mint leaves. Serve hot, with a side of boiled vegetables or a cup of boiled rice.

Chili-Lime Chicken Kabobs (for 8 servings)

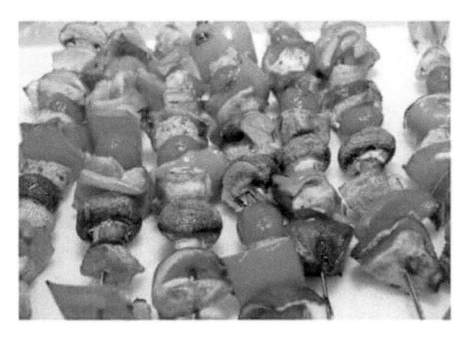

Ingredients:

- 2 pounds of chicken breasts, boneless and skinless, cut into 1 and a ½ inch pieces

- Fresh lime juice from 2 large limes

- 2 tablespoons of red wine vinegar

- 6 tablespoons of olive oil

- 1 teaspoon of garlic powder

- 1 teaspoon of onion powder

- 1 teaspoon paprika

- 2 teaspoons of chili powder

- Cayenne pepper to taste

- Salt and Pepper to taste

Preparation Time: 15 minutes + 1 hour

Cooking Time: 15 minutes

Total time: 1 hour and 30 minutes

Method:

- Whisk the lime juice, olive oil, and vinegar together in a bowl until well mixed. Add the chili powder, onion powder, garlic powder, paprika, cayenne pepper, salt and black pepper, and mix well.

- Place the chicken pieces in a baking dish along with the whisked sauce, and stir so that all the chicken pieces are well covered with the sauce. Cover the baking dish and marinate in the refrigerator for 1 to 1 and a half hour.

- Grease the grill with oil, butter or cooking spray. Preheat the grill on medium to high heat.

- Thread the chicken pieces onto wooden skewers, well coated with marinade. Discard the rest of the marinade.

- Grill the skewers and cook the chicken pieces for 10 to 15 minutes, continuously turning so that the pieces are grilled well all over. Cook till the chicken juices drain and run clear, and the chicken is white and brownish. Serve with mint sauce, pasta, or a bed of egg-fried rice. Other vegetables such as tomatoes, cucumber, mushrooms, capsicum, etc., can also be threaded between the chicken pieces onto the skewers, grilled, and served.

Fish Fillets Italiano (for 8 servings)

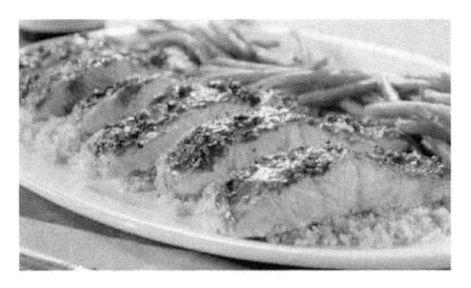

Ingredients:

- 2 pound cod fillets

- 4 tablespoons of olive oil

- 1 cup of dry white wine

- 2 onions, thinly sliced

- 4 cloves of garlic, minced

- 2 tablespoons of fresh parsley, chopped

- 1 cup black olives, pitted and sliced

- 2 cans of tomatoes, diced or 28 ounces of diced tomatoes

Preparation Time: 10 minutes

Cooking Time: 15 minutes

<u>Total time:</u> 25 minutes

<u>Method:</u>

- In a frying pan or large iron skillet, heat oil over medium to high heat. Sauté the onions and garlic in the olive oil until light brown and soft.

- In the fried onions and garlic, add the chopped tomatoes, wine, olives, and parsley, and stir well. Simmer for 5 minutes.

- Place the cod fillets in the sauce, and simmer for another 5 minutes, till the fish turns soft and white.

- Move the fillets and sauce to a serving dish, garnish with chopped mint leaves. Serve with a bed of boiled rice or cooked pasta.

Chickpea Curry (for 8 servings)

Ingredients:

- 2 cans or 15 ounces of garbanzo beans

- 1 cup fresh cilantro, chopped

- 2 tablespoons of vegetable oil

- 2 cloves of garlic, minced

- 2 onions, thinly sliced or minced

- 1 teaspoon of ground turmeric

- 1 teaspoon of cayenne pepper

- 2 teaspoons of ginger root, fresh and finely chopped

- 6 cloves, whole

- 2 large sticks of cinnamon, 2 to 3 inches long, crushed

- 1 teaspoon of ground cumin

- 1 teaspoon of ground coriander

- Salt to taste

Preparation Time: 10 minutes

Cooking Time: 30 minutes

Total time: 40 minutes

Method:

- In a large frying pan or deep iron skillet, heat oil over medium to high heat, and fry the onions until opaque, slightly brown and tender.

- To the onions, add the minced garlic, ginger, whole cloves, cinnamon, coriander, cumin, turmeric powder, cayenne powder, and salt, and stir well. Cook for 1 minute over medium to high heat, stirring constantly. Mix in the garbanzo beans along with the canned liquid. Cook over heat, stirring constantly till all ingredients are well blended and the sauce is heated through.

- Remove pan from heat. Stir in the chopped cilantro. Serve hot, garnish with chopped cilantro or chopped mint leaves. Serve on a bed of boiled rice.

Beef Pot Roast (for 8 servings)

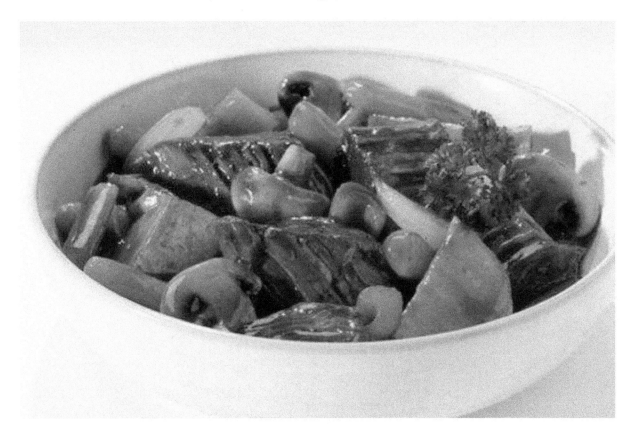

Ingredients:

- 4 pounds of boneless chuck roast

- 2 teaspoons of olive oil

- 1 onion, chopped

- 2 bay leaves

- 2 cloves of garlic, minced

- 1 teaspoon of salt

- ½ teaspoon of freshly ground black pepper

Preparation Time: 20 minutes

Cooking Time: 2 hours

Total time: 2 hours and 20 minutes

Method:

- Preheat an oven to 325 degrees Fahrenheit or 165 degrees Celsius.

- Over medium to high heat, place a heavy Dutch oven on top of the stove. Heat the oil in the Dutch oven, and add the meat. Sear the meat in the pan for 4 to 5 minutes on all sides, using tongs to turn the meat.

- Remove the cooked meat from the pan. Add onions, garlic, and bay leaves to the pan, and sprinkle with salt and pepper. Return the meat to the pan, placing it on top of the other ingredients. Sprinkle crushed bay leaves on the top of the meat pieces, and cover the Dutch oven.

- Bake this dish in the oven for 30 minutes. After that, reduce the heat of the oven to 300 degrees Fahrenheit or 150 degrees Celsius, and cook for another 1 and a ½ hours.

- After this is done, move the roast to a plate, and rest for 10 to 15 minutes to drain all the liquid and unwanted juices from the chicken. Move to a platter, and slice into pieces thick enough to serve. Top the roast with the onions and gravy, and garnish with a piece of celery or chopped mint leaves. Serve hot.

Porcupines (for 10 servings)

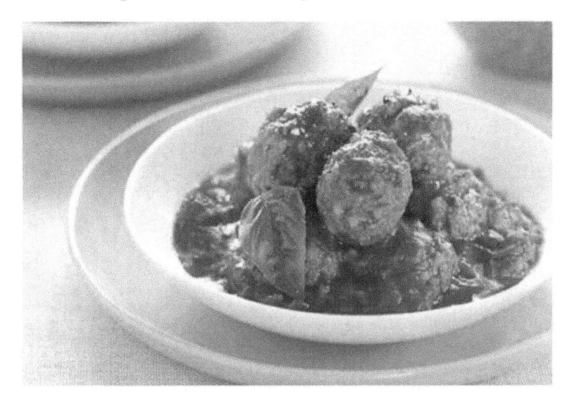

Ingredients:

- 2 pounds of ground beef, lean cut with fat trimmed

- 1 cup of white rice, uncooked

- 2 cans of tomato sauce, or 30 ounces of tomato sauce

- 3 cups of water

- 2 large onions, chopped

- ½ teaspoon ground black pepper

- 2 teaspoons of salt

- 1 teaspoon of celery salt

- ¼ teaspoon of garlic powder

  <u>Preparation Time:</u> 30 minutes

  <u>Cooking Time:</u> 1 hour

  <u>Total time:</u> 1 hour and 30 minutes

  <u>Method:</u>

- Preheat an over to 350 degrees Fahrenheit or 175 degrees Celsius.

- In a bowl, mix together the ground beef, uncooked rice, chopped onions and 1 cup of water. Add salt, celery salt, pepper, and garlic powder to the beef and mix well.

- Using wet hands, make meatballs out of the ground beef, about 1 to 2 inches thick, all of even size.

- In a large iron skillet, add the meatballs and cook well for 3-4 minutes, or till brown, stirring to cook all sides evenly. Drain the fat from the meatballs onto the pan.

- In a baking dish, mix together 2 cups of water and the tomato sauce. Add the browned meatballs to the sauce, mixing well with a wooden spoon to ensure all the meatballs are covered.

- Cover the baking dish, and bake in the preheated oven for 45 to 50 minutes. Remove the lid, and then cook for another 15 minutes. Garnish with chopped mind leaves or a stalk of celery, and on a bed of boiled rice. Serve hot.

Grilled Rock Lobster Tails (for 8 servings)

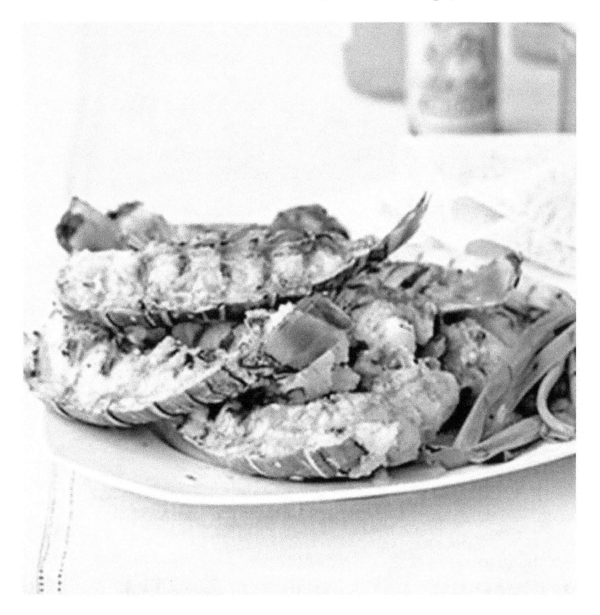

Ingredients:

- 8 rock lobster tails, or 40 ounces of rock lobster tails

- 4 tablespoons of lemon juice

- 2 cups of olive oil

- ½ teaspoon of white pepper

- ½ teaspoon of garlic powder

- 4 teaspoons of salt

- 4 teaspoons of paprika

  Preparation Time: 15 minutes

  Cooking Time: 13 minutes

  Total time: 28 minutes

  Method:

- Preheat a grill at high heat, and grease with cooking spray, butter or oil.

- In a small bowl, add the lemon juice, and slowly mix in the olive oil, using a whisk to combine. Add the white pepper, garlic powder, paprika and salt, and whisk to combine.

- Using a large knife, divide the lobster tails lengthwise. Rub the prepared marinade on the flesh on the inside of the lobster tail.

- On the greased grill grate, place the lobster tails, flesh side on the grill and the other side facing upwards. Cook for 12 to 13 minutes on both sides equally. Baste with marinade every few minutes. When the lobster has been cooked for adequate time, it will be opaque, slightly brown, tender, yet firm to the touch, it should be removed from the heat.

- Serve the lobster hot. Garnish with chopped mint leaves or chopped basil leaves. Serve with a side of boiled vegetables, boiled rice, or a mint dip sauce.

Lentils and Spinach_(for 8 servings)

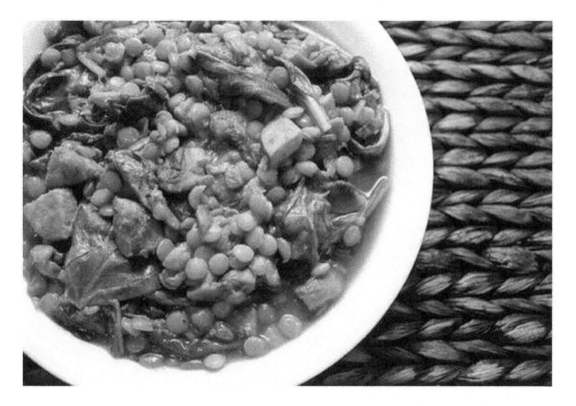

Ingredients:

* 1 cup of lentils

* 2 packs or 20 ounces of frozen spinach

* 4 cups of water

* 2 tablespoons of vegetable oil

* 6 cloves of garlic, minced

* 4 white onions, halved and slices into rings

* 4 cloves of garlic, crushed

* 2 teaspoons of ground cumin

- 2 teaspoons of salt

- Black pepper to taste, freshly ground

  <u>Preparation Time:</u> 10 minutes

  <u>Cooking Time:</u> 55 minutes

  <u>Total time:</u> 1 hour and 5 minutes

  <u>Method:</u>

- In an iron skillet or iron pan, heat oil over medium to high heat. Sauté the onions for around 10 minutes, or until the onions begin to turn golden or light brown. Add the minced garlic and sauté for another minute till the garlic is also light brown.

- In a saucepan, add the water and lentils, and boil the mixture. Cover the pan, and on low heat, simmer for 35 minutes, till the lentils are firm but soft.

- Following the package directions, cook the spinach in the microwave or simply boil the spinach leaves for a minute in boiling water.

- In a saucepan, add the boiled and drained lentils, sautéed garlic and onions, spinach, salt and cumin. Cover, and simmer everything for around 10 minutes till all the ingredients are heated through. Add pepper and extra garlic to the mixture, according to taste.

- Serve hot. Garnish with chopped mint leaves or a stalk of celery. Serve with boiled vegetables or boiled rice.

Mushroom Risotto (for 8 servings)

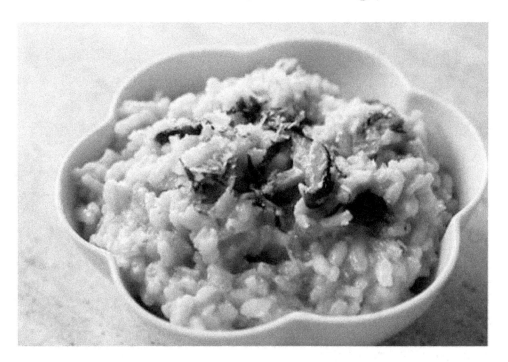

Ingredients:

- 3 cups fresh mushrooms, thinly sliced

- 2 cups of whole milk

- 2 cups of rice, any gluten free variety, uncooked

- ½ cup of heavy cream

- 2 cups grated Parmesan cheese

- 2 tablespoons olive oil

- 4 large onions, finely chopped

- 10 cups vegetable stalk

- 2 cloves of garlic, crushed

- 2 teaspoons butter

- 2 teaspoons fresh parsley, minced

- 2 teaspoons fresh celery, minced

- Salt and Pepper to taste

  <u>Preparation Time:</u> 10 minutes

  <u>Cooking Time:</u> 35 minutes

  <u>Total time:</u> 45 minutes

  <u>Method:</u>

- Heat olive oil in a large pan over medium to high heat. Sauté the garlic and onions till tender and lightly browned. Remove garlic from the pan, and stir in parsley, celery, salt and pepper. Cook on heat until the celery is soft and tender. Add the mushrooms, and cook on low heat till mushrooms are soft.

- Add milk, cream and rice to the pan, and stir well with a wooden spoon. Simmer for a few minutes. Add the vegetable stock, one cup at a time, until it is well absorbed and reduced.

- Once the rice is soft, tender and has finished cooking, add the Parmesan cheese and butter to the pan. Move to a serving dish, and serve hot.

Scott Ure's Clams and Garlic (for 4 servings)

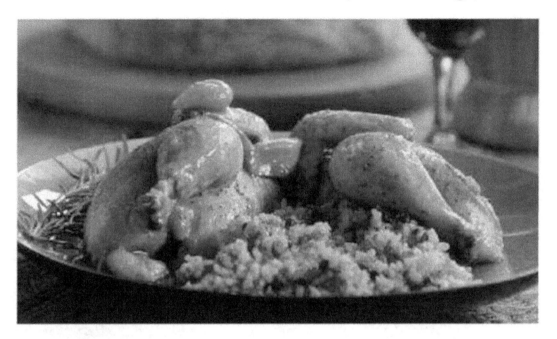

Ingredients:

- 50 small clams in the shell, well scrubbed

- 2 tablespoons butter

- ½ cup of fresh parsley, chopped

- 6 cloves garlic, minced

- 2 tablespoons of extra virgin olive oil

- 1 cup of white wine

  Preparation Time: 25 minutes

  Cooking Time: 25 minutes

  Total time: 50 minutes

<u>Method:</u>

- Wash clams and scrub well to remove dirt and sand.

- In a large pot, heat olive oil over medium to high heat. Sauté the garlic for one minute or till tender. Add white wine to the pot, and boil till wine is reduced to half its volume.

- Add the clams to the pot and cover. Simmer on low heat till the clamshells begin to open. Add the butter, cover again, and cook till most clams open. Discard the ones that do not.

- Move the sauce and the clams to a large serving bowl. Garnish with chopped parsley. Serve with crusty Italian bread or on a bed of pasta or boiled rice. Serve hot.

Rosemary Braised Lamb Shanks (for 4 servings)

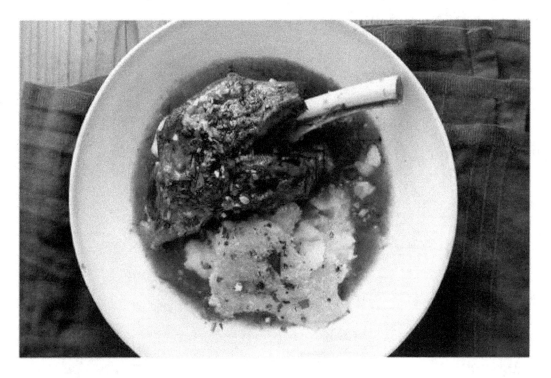

Ingredients:

- 4 lamb shanks, lean cut with fat trimmed

- 1 and a ½ tablespoon of olive oil

- 1 can or 20 ounces of whole peeled tomatoes with juice

- 1 large onions, chopped

- 6 cloves of garlic, minced

- 2 large carrots, cut into ¼ inch round pieces

- ¾ bottle of red wine, or 550 ml of red wine

- ¾ can or 7 ounces of beef broth

- ¾ can or 7 ounces of condensed chicken broth

- 3 teaspoons fresh rosemary, chopped

- 1 teaspoon fresh thyme, chopped

- Salt and Pepper to taste

  <u>Preparation Time:</u> 30 minutes

  <u>Cooking Time:</u> 2 hours

  <u>Total time:</u> 2 hours and 30 minutes

  <u>Method:</u>

- Rub the lamb shanks with salt and pepper. Heat oil in a large heavy pot over medium to high heat. Cooking only a few shanks at a time, cook in the pot, using tongs to flip, and brown the shanks all over. Cook for about 8 minutes, and then drain the oil from the shanks by letting them rest on a plate.

- In the same pot, add garlic, carrots and onions, and over medium to high heat, sauté for 10 minutes, or till golden brown. Add the tomatoes, chicken broth, beef broth and wine, and stir well using a wooden spoon. Season the sauce with thyme and rosemary and stir well.

- Add the shanks to the pot, pressing on them with a wooden spoon to cover them completely with the sauce. Cover the pot and bring the liquid to a boil, and then lower heat and simmer for about 2 hours, till the meat is soft and tender.

- Remove the cover from the pot, and simmer for another 20 minutes. Remove the shanks from the pot and set on a serving plate. Thicken and reduce the sauces in the pot until of good thick consistency, for about 15 minutes. Pour the sauce over the shanks. Garnish with chopped fresh parsley or mint leaves. Serve with crispy bread or boiled rice.

Grilled Sea Bass (for 12 servings)

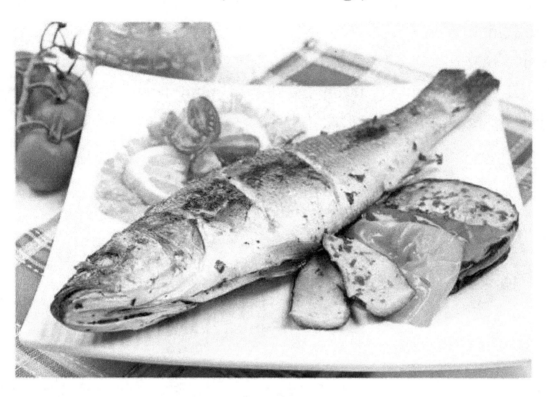

Ingredients:

- 4 pounds of sea bass

- 6 tablespoons butter

- 2 large cloves of garlic, chopped

- ½ teaspoon garlic powder

- ½ teaspoon onion powder

- ½ teaspoon paprika

- 2 tablespoons of Italian flat leaf parsley, chopped

- 3 tablespoons of extra virgin olive oil

- Sea salt to taste

- Lemon pepper to taste

  <u>Preparation Time:</u> 20 minutes

  <u>Cooking Time:</u> 20 minutes

  <u>Total time:</u> 40 minutes

  <u>Method:</u>

- Preheat grill on high heat.

- Mix together the onion powder, garlic powder, paprika, sea salt and lemon pepper in a bowl. Mix well, and rub the seasoning onto the washed and dried sea bass.

- In a small saucepan, add butter, parsley and garlic, and melt and cook over medium heat. When butter has fully melted, remove the pan from heat, mix well, and set the pan aside to rest.

- Grease the grill using butter, oil or cooking spray. Grill the fish for 7 minutes on each side, flipping the fish using tongs. Drizzle with butter to prevent sticking and add flavor. Cook till the fish is soft and very tender. Drizzle with olive oil before serving. Serve hot with boiled vegetables or tartar sauce (made from gluten free ingredients).

Harvest Rice Dish (for 6 servings)

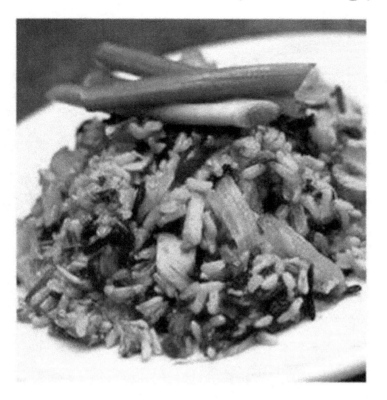

Ingredients:

- ½ cup of brown rice, uncooked

- ½ cup of wild rice, uncooked

- ½ cup of silvered almonds

- 2/3 cup fresh mushrooms, thinly sliced

- 3 onions, sliced into thin wedges

- 2 tablespoons butter

- 1 cup dried cranberries

- 2 cups of chicken broth

- 1 tablespoon brown sugar

- ½ teaspoon orange zest

- Salt and Pepper to taste

  Preparation Time: 15 minutes

  Cooking Time: 1 hour and 30 minutes

  Total time: 1 hour and 45 minutes

  Method:

- Preheat the oven to 350 degrees Fahrenheit or 175 degrees Celsius. Put almonds on an ungreased baking tray and toast in the oven for 6 to 8 minutes.

- In a saucepan, mix the two types of rice and the broth, and boil. After bringing it to boil, cover, and simmer on low heat for 40 to 45 minutes till the broth has been absorbed and the rice is tender.

- In a pan, melt butter over medium to high heat. Sauté the onions and brown sugar till onions are translucent and soft, and butter has been absorbed. Reduce heat to low, and cook onions for 15 to 20 minutes till they have caramelized.

- Add the cranberries and mushrooms to the pan. Stir well. Cover the pan, and cook for 10 to 15 minutes or till the berries start to absorb liquid. Mix in the orange zest and almonds, and then fold in the whole mixture into the cooked rice. Add salt and pepper to taste, and serve warm.

Quick Chicken and Wine (for 6 servings)

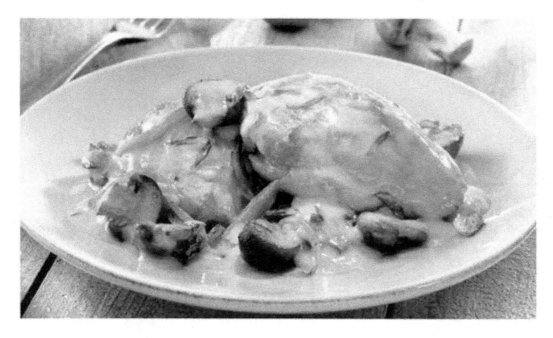

Ingredients:

- 4 chicken breast halves, skinless, boneless and cut into thin strips

- ½ cup white wine

- 4 tablespoons of butter

- ½ cup of Parmesan cheese, crumbled

- 2 eggs, beaten

- 1 teaspoon of salt

- 1 teaspoon of pepper

Preparation Time: 10 minutes

Cooking Time: 30 minutes

Total time: 40 minutes

Method:

- Arrange three plates and a bowl on the counter. On one plate, sprinkle the mixture of salt and pepper. On the next plate, cut each breast half into three pieces, and in the third, sprinkle the crumbled Parmesan cheese. Beat the eggs well with a whisk in a bowl.

- First season the chicken with the salt and pepper, then dip in eggs, and coat with Parmesan cheese. Repeat for all pieces. You may need to adjust the quantity of Parmesan, eggs and seasoning to be adequate for all chicken pieces.

- In a frying pan, melt butter over medium to high heat. Add the chicken pieces, stir and cook well, till tender and golden brown.

- Add the wine, cover the pan, and simmer on low heat for around 20-25 minutes. Once done, move the chicken to a serving platter, and serve on a bed of pasta, boiled rice, boiled vegetables or crusty bread.

Baked Tilapia in Garlic and Olive Oil (for 8 servings)

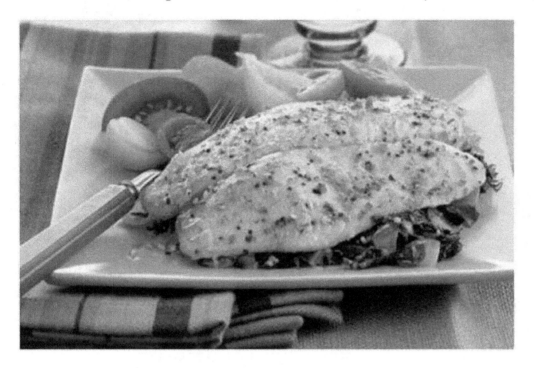

Ingredients:

- 8 fillets or 8 ounces of tilapia

- 6 tablespoons of olive oil

- 2 onions, chopped

- 8 cloves garlic, crushed

- ½ teaspoon of cayenne pepper

Preparation Time: 5 minutes

Cooking Time: 30 minutes

Total time: 1 hour and 35 minutes

Method:

- Rub the crushed garlic onto the fish fillets, and coat them well with olive oil in a shallow dish. Place the chopped onions over the fish. Cover the dish, and marinate overnight.

- Before cooking, preheat the oven to 350 degrees Fahrenheit or 175 degrees Celsius.

- Grease a baking dish with butter or oil, and move the fish along with the garlic, onions, and olive oil into the dish. Sprinkle the cayenne pepper on to. Bake for 30-35 minutes till brown and tender. Serve with tartar sauce, or crust Italian bread.

Maple Glazed Ribs (for 6 servings)

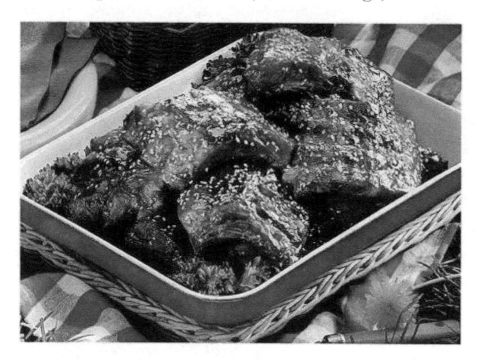

Ingredients:

- 3 pounds of baby back pork ribs

- 2 tablespoons of ketchup

- ¾ cup maple syrup

- 1 tablespoon Worcestershire sauce

- 2 tablespoons brown sugar

- ½ teaspoon mustard powder

- 1 tablespoon cider vinegar

- ½ teaspoon salt

Preparation Time: 15 minutes + 2 hours

Cooking Time: 1 hour and 25 minutes

Total time: 3 hours and 40 minutes

Method:

- Place the ribs in water in a pot. Cover and simmer on low heat for 1 hour, or till meat is tender. Drain, and move ribs to a shallow dish.

- Stir the maple syrup, ketchup, vinegar, brown sugar, mustard powder, Worcestershire sauce, and salt in a saucepan. Bring to a low boil and cook for 5 minutes, stirring constantly. Cool the sauce, pour it over the ribs, and refrigerate for 2 hours.

- Preheat the grill on High, grease with oil or butter. Cook the ribs for 20 minutes on the grate, on both sides, basting frequently, till browned and glazed.

- Boil the leftover marinade and thicken, pour over ribs in a servings platter. Garnish with chopped parsley, serve hot, with crusty bread, or boiled rice

CHAPTER 8: GLUTEN-FREE RECIPES FOR SNACKS

Quinoa and Black Beans (for 10 servings)

Ingredients:

- 1 onion, chopped

- 3 cloves garlic, chopped

- ¼ teaspoon cayenne peppers

- 1 cup frozen corn kernels

- ½ cup fresh cilantro, chopped

- 1 teaspoon ground cumin

- 1 and ½ cups vegetable broth

- 1 teaspoon vegetable oil

- ¾ cup quinoa

- 1 cans (15 ounces) black beans, rinsed and drained

- Salt and ground black pepper, to taste

Preparation time: 15 minutes

Cooking time: 35 minutes

Total Time: 50 minutes

Method:

- Heat oil in a wok or a non-stick pan over medium heat, and cook and stir the onion and garlic for around 10 minutes till lightly browned.

- Mix the quinoa into the onion mixture and add the vegetable broth. Stir, and season with cumin, cayenne pepper, salt and pepper.

- Boil the mixture, then cover, reduce the heat and simmer the mixture until the quinoa is tender and the broth is absorbed by the quinoa. This will take around 20 minutes.

- Stir the frozen corn kernels into the quinoa mixture, and simmer until the whole mixture is heated through, which will take around 5 minutes.

- At the end, mix the black beans and cilantro, and serve. This dish can be eaten as a snack, appetizer, or as a side dish to a main dish.

Vegetarian Chickpea Sandwich Filling (for 6 servings)

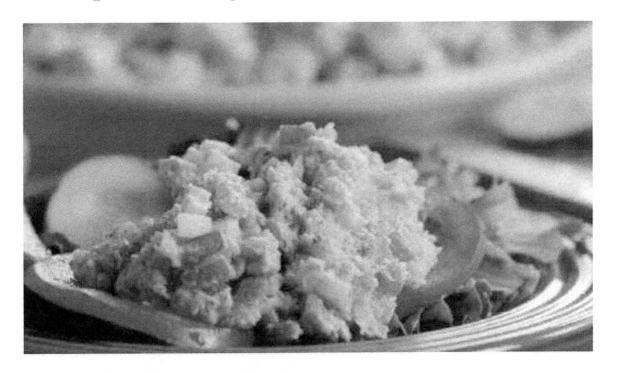

Ingredients:

- 2 cans or 40 ounces of garbanzo beans

- 1 onion, chopped

- 2 tablespoons lemon juice

- 2 tablespoons mayonnaise

- 2 stalks of celery, chopped

- 2 teaspoons of dried dill weed

- Salt and Pepper to taste

Preparation Time: 20 minutes

Total time: 20 minutes

Method:

- Drain and rinse the garbanzo beans. Put into a bowl and mash well using a masher or fork. Mix in the chopped onions, celery, lemon juice, mayonnaise, dill, salt and pepper to taste. Refrigerate, and use in bread rolls or in sandwiches with tomato ketchup.

Broiled Scallops (for 6 servings)

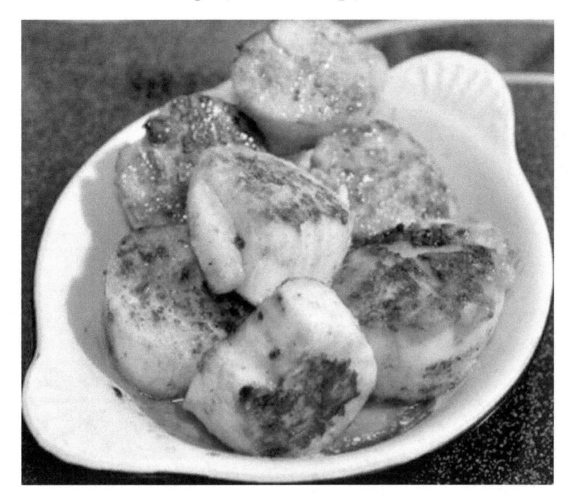

Ingredients:

- 3 pounds of bay scallops

- 4 tablespoons lemon juice

- 4 tablespoons butter

- 2 tablespoons garlic salt

Preparation Time: 5 minutes

Cooking Time: 10 minutes

Total time: 15 minutes

<u>Method:</u>

- Turn on the broiler. Rinse scallops and in a baking pan, mix in melted butter, lemon juice, and garlic salt.

- Broil the scallops for 8 to 10 minutes until they turn golden brown. Remove from the oven, serve with melted butter, crispy bread or boiled vegetables.

Roasted Brussels Sprouts (for 6 servings)

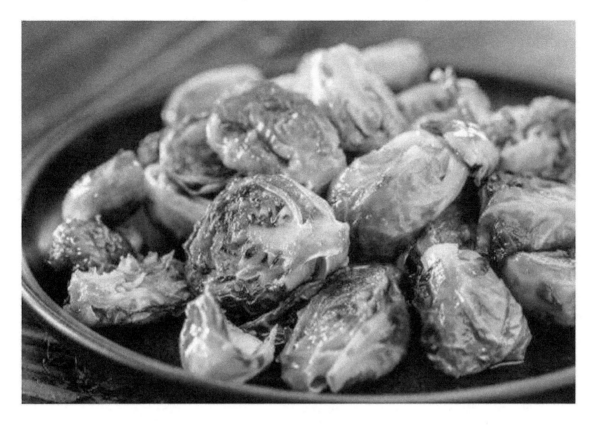

Ingredients:

- 1 and a ½ pounds Brussels sprouts, yellow leaves and ends removed

- 1 teaspoon kosher salt

- 3 tablespoons olive oil

- ½ teaspoon freshly ground black pepper

  <u>Preparation Time:</u> 15 minutes

  <u>Cooking Time:</u> 45 minutes

  <u>Total time:</u> 1 hour

  <u>Method:</u>

- Preheat oven to 400 degrees Fahrenheit or 205 degrees Celsius.

- Place the Brussels sprouts, kosher salt, pepper and olive oil in an airtight plastic bag. Seal and shake.

- Pour ingredients onto baking sheet, bake in oven for 40 to 45 minutes, or till sprouts are dark brown. Shake pan occasionally to ensure equal browning. Season with salt and pepper, and serve hot.

Tequila Shrimp (for 12 servings)

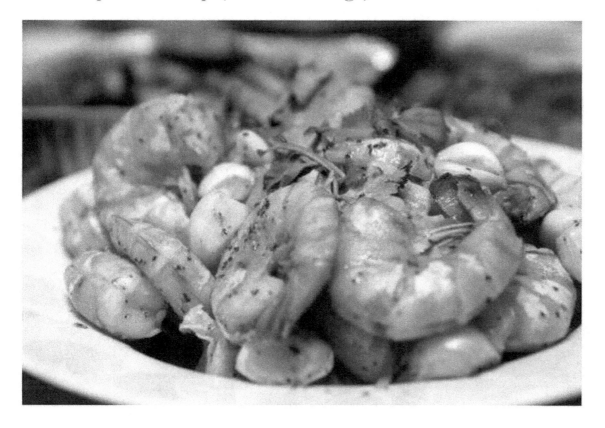

Ingredients:

- 3 pounds shrimp, peeled and deveined

- 8 cloves garlic, crushed

- 4 tablespoons unsalted butter

- 1 cup tequila

- 1 cup fresh cilantro, chopped

- Salt and Pepper to taste

Preparation Time: 10 minutes

Cooking Time: 10 minutes

Total time: 20 minutes

Method:

- In a large pan, melt butter and sauté garlic till golden brown. Add shrimp to pan, cook for 3 to 4 minutes on both sides evenly.

- Add the tequila, cilantro, salt and pepper and cook for another 2 minutes. Serve hot with accompanying dip.

Authentic Huevos Rancheros (for 8 servings)

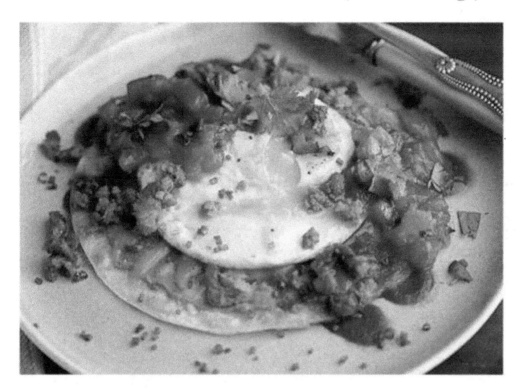

Ingredients:

- 16 slices bacon, cooked and crushed

- 8 corn tortillas, 6 inches each

- 4 tablespoons vegetable oil

- 2 teaspoons butter

- 8 eggs

- 2 cups Cheddar cheese, shredded

- 1 cup salsa

- 2 cups refried beans with green chilies

Preparation Time: 10 minutes

Cooking Time: 10 minutes

Method:

- Heat oil over medium to high heat in a pan or iron skillet. Fry tortillas, one at a time, till firm. Drain to grease.

- Mix the refried beans and butter in the microwave dish and cook in the microwave till well heated.

- Fry eggs in a pan.

- Place tortilla onto a plate. Spread a layer of beans on them. Add the cheese, a fried egg to each, crumbled bacon, and salsa. Serve hot or cold.

Feta and Olive Meatballs (for 8 servings)

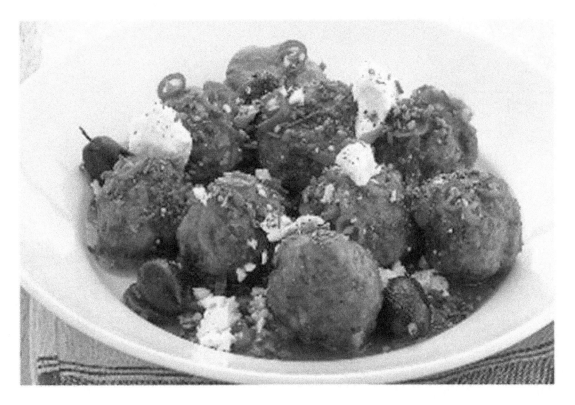

Ingredients:

- 1 pound of lamb, ground

- 1 onion, finely chopped

- ½ cup green olives, chopped

- 2 eggs

- ½ cup fresh parsley, chopped

- ½ cup feta cheese, crumbled

- 1 teaspoon Italian seasoning

Preparation Time: 10 minutes

Cooking Time: 10 minutes

Total time: 20 minutes

Method:

- Preheat your oven's broiler.

- Mix the ground lamb, parsley, onion, green olives, eggs, feta cheese and Italian seasoning well in a bowl. Using your hands, shape the mixture into 16 round meatballs, and place on greased baking tray two inches apart.

- Broil the meatballs for around 3 minutes until they are soft, tender and firm in their shape, and browned from the top, then using tongs, turn over and broil on the other side too. Serve hot, with sauce.

Garlic Crab Legs (for 8 servings)

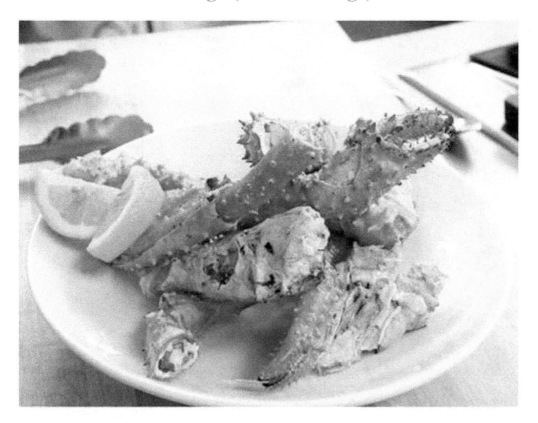

Ingredients:

- 3 and a ½ pounds of Alaskan King crab legs with shell intact

- 6 ears of fresh corn

- 1 and ½ cups butter

- 1 teaspoons garlic, minced

- 1/8 teaspoon red pepper flakes, crushed

- 1 teaspoon Old Bay Seasoning

Preparation Time: 10 minutes

Cooking Time: 25 minutes

Total time: 35 minutes

<u>Method:</u>

- In a large stockpot, bring the water to a boil, add in the crab legs and corn, and boil them in water till the corn is tender and firm, and the crab legs are soft, opaque and flaky. Drain crab legs and corn once done.

- Melt butter in a saucepan, and add in margarine, red pepper, old bay seasoning, and garlic, and mix well. Add the crab and corn, and sauté them in the seasoning for 5 to 10 minutes. Serve hot. Cut slits into crab leg shells to make access to meat easier.

Indian Style Seekh Kebab (for 8 servings)

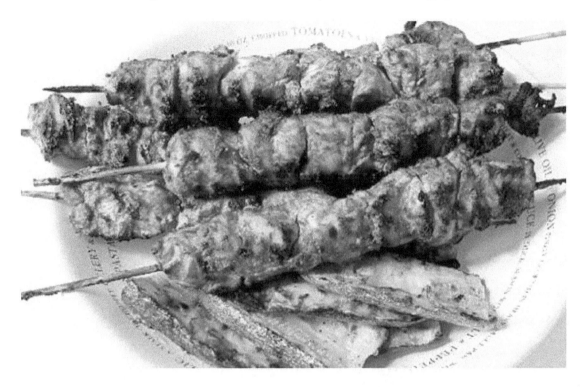

<u>Ingredients:</u>

- 2 pounds ground lamb, meat trimmed

- 2 onions, finely chopped

- ½ cup cilantro, finely chopped

- ½ cup mint leaves, finely chopped

- 2 teaspoons ground cumin

- 1 tablespoon ginger paste

- 1 tablespoon green chili paste

- 2 teaspoons ground coriander

- ½ cup vegetable oil

- 2 teaspoons paprika

- 1 teaspoon cayenne pepper

- 2 teaspoons salt

  Preparation Time: 15 minutes + 2 hours

  Cooking Time: 10 minutes

  Total time: 2 hours and 25 minutes

  Method:

- Mix ground lamb, onions, Chile paste, ginger paste, cilantro, mint, cumin, coriander, and cayenne, paprika and salt in a bowl. Cover and refrigerate for 2 hours.

- Take one cup of the mixture and mold to form an even sausage shape around skewers. Do the same for all till mixture finished.

- Preheat grill at high heat. Grease with butter or oil, Arrange kebabs on the grill, and cook for 10 minutes, turning skewers every few minutes to brown evenly. Serve hot with yoghurt and mint sauce.

Serbian Cevapcici (for 8 servings)

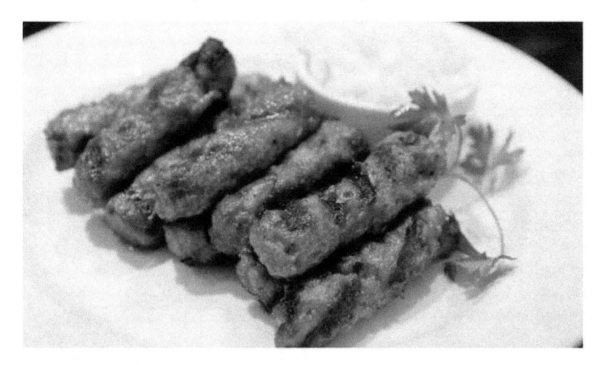

Ingredients:

- 3 pounds ground pork

- 2 pounds ground lean beef

- 1 pound ground lamb

- 2 egg whites

- 8 cloves garlic, minced

- 2 teaspoons salt

- 2 teaspoons baking soda

- 4 teaspoons ground black pepper

- 1 teaspoon paprika

- 2 teaspoons cayenne pepper

  <u>Preparation Time:</u> 10 minutes

  <u>Cooking Time:</u> 30 minutes

  <u>Total time:</u> 40 minutes

  <u>Method:</u>

- Preheat a grill on medium to low heat.

- Combine the ground beef, pork, lamb, egg whites, garlic, salt, black pepper, cayenne pepper, baking soda and paprika well in a bowl. Combine well with wet hands, and mold into 3 inch sausages ¾ inches think.

- Grease grilling surface with oil. Grill sausages till cooked through for 30 minutes, till browned, turning every few minutes. Serve with yoghurt mint sauce.

CHAPTER 9: GLUTEN-FREE RECIPES FOR APPETIZERS

STUFFED PEPPERS (FOR 6 SERVINGS)

BUFFALO CHICKEN WINGS (MAKES 24 WINGS)

YUMMY ROLL UPS (FOR 10 SERVINGS)

HUMMUS (MAKES 2 CUPS)

GRILLED SHRIMP SCAMPI (FOR 12 SERVINGS)

GRILLED PORTOBELLO MUSHROOMS (FOR 6 SERVINGS)

CRAB STUFFED MUSHROOMS (FOR 6 SERVINGS)

BACON AND DATE APPETIZER (FOR 12 SERVINGS)

ASPARAGUS WRAPPED IN CRISP PROSCIUTTO (FOR 16 SERVINGS)

ARTICHOKE SALSA (MAKES 2 AND A ½ CUPS)

Stuffed Peppers (for 6 servings)

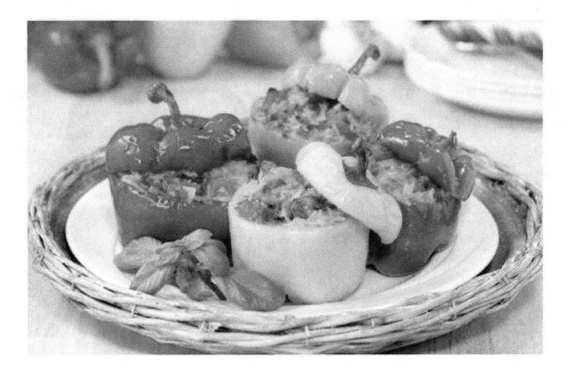

Ingredients:

- ½ pound of ground beef

- ¼ cup of uncooked white rice (or any other gluten free rice variety)

- ½ cup water

- 1 can or 4 ounces of tomato sauce

- ½ tablespoon of Worcestershire sauce

- 3 green bell peppers

- ½ teaspoon Italian seasoning

- A few pinches garlic powder

- A few pinches of onion powder

- Salt and Pepper to taste

  Preparation Time: 20 minutes

  Cooking time: 1 hour

  Total time: 1hour and 20 minutes

  Method:

- Preheat the oven to 350 degrees Fahrenheit or 175 degrees Celsius.

- In a saucepan, add the rice and water and bring the mixture to a boil. Then reduce the heat, cover, and cook for 20 minutes. In a greased pan or an iron skillet, cook the beef over medium heat until it is evenly browned.

- Remove and discard the tops, seeds and membranes of all of the bell peppers. In a greased baking dish, arrange the peppers with the hollow portions facing upwards.

- Place the browned beef, cooked rice, Worcestershire sauce, 2 ounces tomato sauce, garlic powder, onion powder, salt and pepper in a bowl, and mix well.

- Using a spoon put an equal amount of mixture neatly into each hollowed pepper.

- Mix the leftover 2 ounces of tomato sauce and Italian seasoning in a bowl and pour over the stuffed peppers.

- Bake the peppers for 1 hour in the preheated oven, and baste with sauce every 15 minutes to prevent drying out. Bake till the peppers are tender. Serve warm, as a snack or appetizer.

Buffalo Chicken Wings (makes 24 wings)

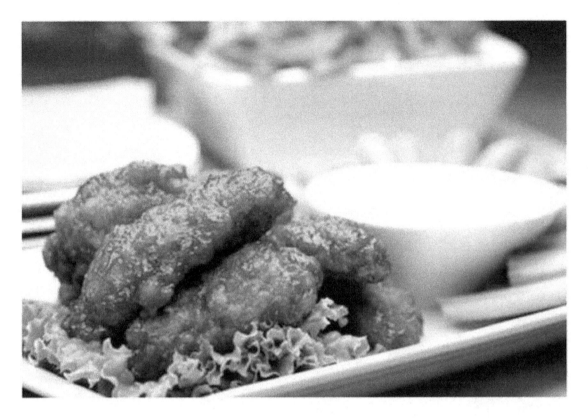

Ingredients:

- 24 chicken wings, tips removed and the wings cut in half at the joint

- 1 liter vegetable oil for deep frying

- 4 tablespoons butter

- 1 tablespoon distilled white vinegar

- 5 tablespoons hot pepper sauce

- Salt and Pepper to taste

  Preparation time: 10 minutes

  Cooking time: 15 minutes

  Total time: 25 minutes

  Method:

- Heat the vegetable oil in a deep fryer, and using thermometer, heat to 375 degrees Fahrenheit or 190 degrees Celsius.

- Deep-fry the chicken wings in oil until brown, for about 10 minutes. Remove the chicken from the fryer and drain.

- Melt butter in a large pan, or an iron skillet. Add the hot pepper sauce and vinegar to the butter, and season with salt and pepper, adjusted to taste.

- Add the cooked chicken to the sauce in the skillet and cook over low heat till sauce thickens and starts coating the wings. The longer you allow the wings to simmer in the sauce, the hotter they will be. Serve warm, garnished with mint, as an appetizer.

Yummy Roll ups (for 10 servings)

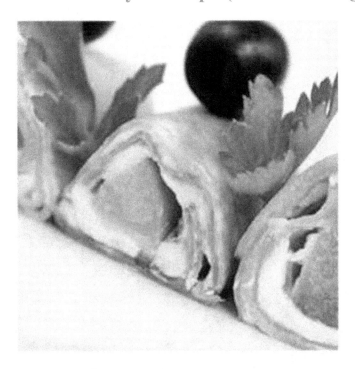

Ingredients:

- 10 slices of cooked ham

- 10 dill pickle spears

- 2 packages or 16 ounces softened cream cheese

  Preparation Time: 10 minutes

  Total Time: 10 minutes

  Method:

- Lay the ham slices flat on a plate and pat them dry using paper towels. Spread the cream cheese on each slice neatly in one uniform layer.

- Put a pickle spear at one end of each of the slices, and roll the slices into cylinders around the spears. Secure with toothpicks and serve cold as appetizers.

Hummus (makes 2 cups)

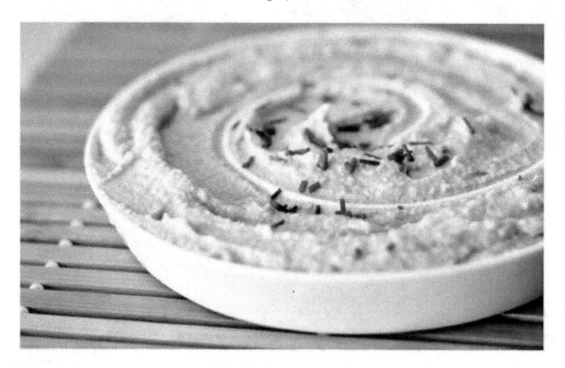

Ingredients:

- 2 cups of canned garbanzo beans

- ¼ cup of lemon juice

- 1/3 cup of tahini

- 2 cloves garlic, cut in half

- 1 tablespoon olive oil

- 1 teaspoon salt

- 1 pinch of paprika

- 1 teaspoon of minced fresh parsley

  <u>Preparation time:</u> 10 minutes

  <u>Total time:</u> 10 minutes

  <u>Method:</u>

- Drain the canned garbanzo beans, and then place them along with garlic, lemon juice, salt and tahini in a food processor or a blender. Blend together into a paste until it is smooth. Move the mixture into a serving bowl.

- Drizzle olive oil on top of the garbanzo bean mixture. Garnish or sprinkle with parsley and paprika, and serve with pita bread or any sort of gluten free bread.

Grilled Shrimp Scampi (for 12 servings)

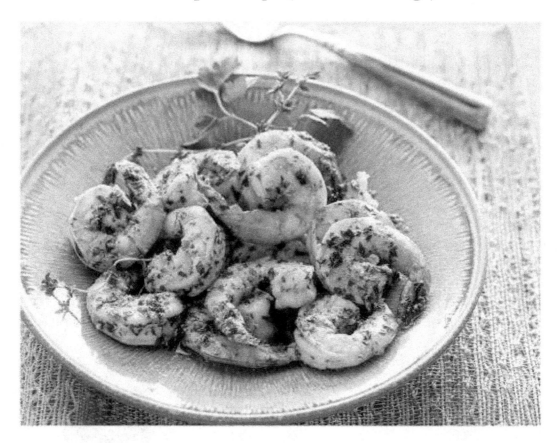

Ingredients:

- 3 pounds of medium shrimp, peeled and deveined

- ½ cup lemon juice

- ½ cup olive oil

- 6 tablespoons of freshly chopped parsley

- 2 tablespoons minced garlic

- Ground black pepper to taste

- Crushed red pepper flakes to taste (optional)

Preparation time: 30 minutes

Cooking time: 6 minutes

Total time: 36 minutes

Method:

- Stir the lemon juice, olive oil, garlic, parsley and black pepper in a large plastic or metal bowl. Season with crushed red chilies, which is optional.

- Add the shrimp to the bowl, and toss in order to coat the shrimp. Marinate in the refrigerator for 30 minutes

- Preheat a grill at high heat. Place the shrimp on skewers, piercing near the tail and the head. Discard the remaining marinade, as it does not need to be used.

- Grease the grill grate using oil or butter. Grill the shrimp on skewers on each side till opaque and light brown, around 2 to 3 minutes per side. Serve warm with parsley or an accompanying dip.

Grilled Portobello Mushrooms (for 6 servings)

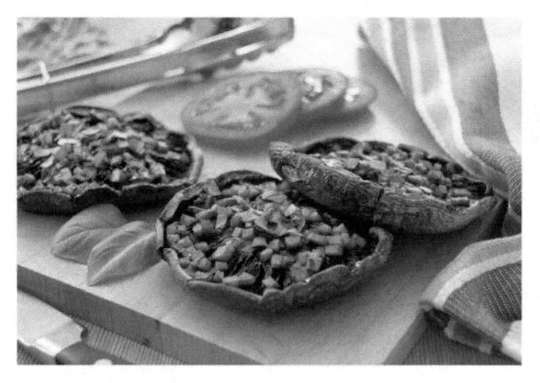

Ingredients:

- 6 Portobello mushrooms

- 6 tablespoons of chopped onion

- 8 cloves of garlic, minced

- ½ cup of canola oil

- 8 tablespoons balsamic vinegar

Preparation time: 1 hour and 10 minutes

Cooking time: 10 minutes

Total time: 1 hour and 20 minutes

Method:

- Clean the mushrooms by washing with water and removing the stems. Place the caps on a plate with the gills facing upwards.

- Combine the vinegar, oil, onion and garlic in a bowl, and mix well. Pour this mixture uniformly over the mushroom caps and let it stand for one hour.

- Preheat a grill to high heat and grease will cooking spray, butter or oil. Grill the mushrooms over the hot grill for 10 minutes. Serve hot.

Crab Stuffed Mushrooms (for 6 servings)

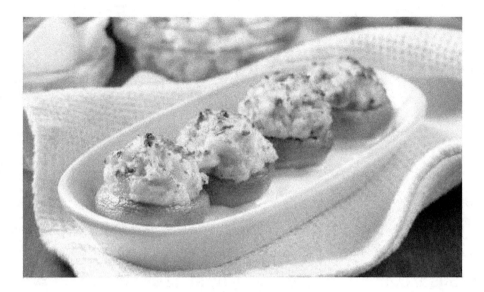

Ingredients:

- 1 pound of fresh mushrooms

- 7 ounces of crabmeat

- ¼ teaspoons of dried oregano

- ¼ teaspoons of dried Lyme

- 5 green onions, thinly sliced

- ¼ cup grated parmesan cheese

- 3 tablespoons grated parmesan cheese

- 1/3 cup mayonnaise

- ¼ teaspoon paprika

- ¼ teaspoon ground savory

- Ground black pepper to taste

Preparation time: 25 minutes

Cooking time: 15 minutes

Total Time: 40 minutes

Method:

- Preheat the oven to 350 degrees Fahrenheit or 175 degrees Celsius.

- Combine the crabmeat, herbs, green onions and pepper in a bowl. Combine ¼ cups of Parmesan cheese and mayonnaise in the bowl and mix till well combined. Refrigerate the mixture till chilled.

- Dry and wipe the mushrooms till clean, and remove the stems. Spoon out the gills and cut off the base of the stem, allowing the inside to become a hollow cup.

- Spoon the refrigerated filling into the mushroom cups, and place them in an ungreased baking dish. Sprinkle the mushroom tops with paprika and 3 tablespoons of Parmesan cheese.

- Bake for 15 minutes. Remove from the oven, and serve hot.

Bacon and Date Appetizer (for 12 servings)

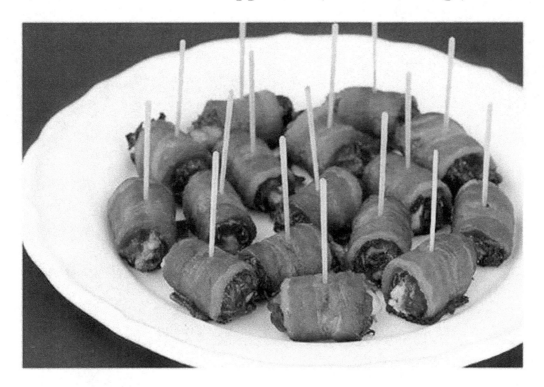

Ingredients:

- 2 packets or 16 ounces of pitted dates

- 2 pounds of bacon, sliced

- 8 ounces of almonds

Preparation time: 30 minutes

Cooking time: 5 minutes

<u>Total Time:</u> 35 minutes

<u>Method:</u>

- Preheat the broiler to a high temperature.

- Slit the dates from the top without cutting into half. Place one almond inside each date, and wrap the dates with bacon slices. Use toothpicks to secure the bacon slices on top of the date.

- Broil the bacon covered dates for 10 minutes, or until the bacon is brown and crisp. Serve warm or cold.

Asparagus wrapped in Crisp Prosciutto (for 16 servings)

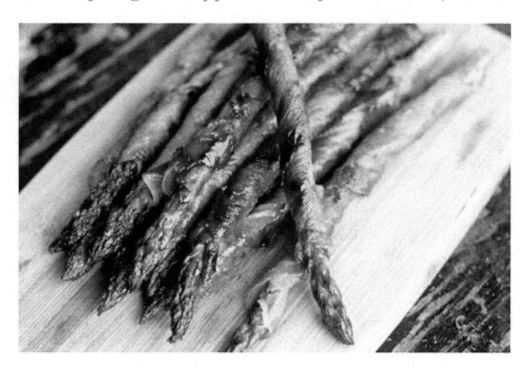

Ingredients:

- 16 slices of prosciutto

- 16 spears fresh asparagus, trimmed

- 1 tablespoon of olive oil

  Preparation time: 5 minutes

  Cooking time: 15 minutes

  Total Time: 20 minutes

  Method:

- Preheat the oven to 450 degrees Fahrenheit or 220 degrees Celsius.

- Line a baking sheet with aluminum foil and coat the foil with olive oil.

- Wrap one slice of prosciutto around each of the asparagus spears, starting at the bottom of the spear and wrapping it around until it reaches the top. Place the wrapped spears on the prepared baking sheet.

- Bake the pears for 5 minutes in the oven. Remove the pan and shake the pan back and forth to turn over the spears. Return to the oven for another 5 minutes and bake till the prosciutto is crisp and the asparagus is tender. Serve hot.

Artichoke Salsa (makes 2 and a ½ cups)

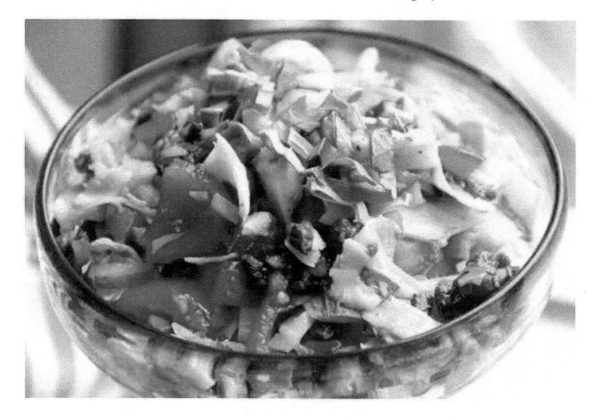

Ingredients:

- 2 jars or 13 ounces of jar marinated artichoke hearts, drained, dried and chopped

- 4 tablespoons of chopped red onion

- 2 tablespoons of chopped garlic

- 4 tablespoons chopped fresh basil

- ½ cup chopped black olives

- 6 roma (plum) tomatoes, chopped

- Salt and Pepper to taste

Preparation time: 15 minutes

Method:

- Mix the artichoke hearts, onions, olives, tomatoes, garlic, salt and pepper in a bowl. Mix well. Serve chilled, with tortilla chips or any made out of gluten free materials.

CHAPTER 10: GLUTEN-FREE RECIPES FOR SALADS

Vietnamese Rice Noodle Salad (for 4 servings)

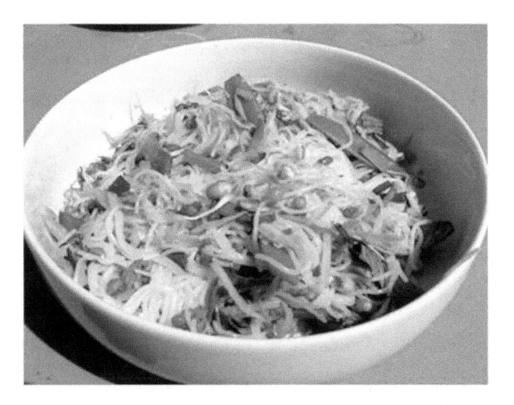

Ingredients:

- ½ jalapeno pepper, seeded and minced

- 5 cloves of garlic

- 1 cup chopped cilantro

- 2 carrots, julienned

- 1 chopped cucumber

- ¼ cup fresh mint, chopped

- 4 leaves napa cabbage

- 4 sprigs fresh mint

- 3 tablespoons vegetarian fish sauce

- 3 tablespoons white sugar

- ¼ cup fresh lime juice

- 1 package (12 ounce) dried rice noodles

- ½ cup unsalted peanuts

  Preparation Time: 15 minutes

  Total time: 15 minutes

  Method:

- Mince the garlic, hot peppers and cilantro, and shift the mixture to a bowl.

- Add fish sauce, lime juice, salt and sugar and to the bowl and mix well. Let the whole thing sit for 5 minutes.

- Boil a large saucepan of salted water, add the rice noodles when the water comes to boil, and cook them for 2 minutes. Drain when boiled, and rinse with cold water to cool.

- Combine the noodles, sauce, and the vegetables (carrots, cucumber, mint, and napa cabbage) in a large bowl. Toss the ingredients, and serve the salad garnished with mint sprigs and peanuts.

Radicchio Salad with Frisee and Apples

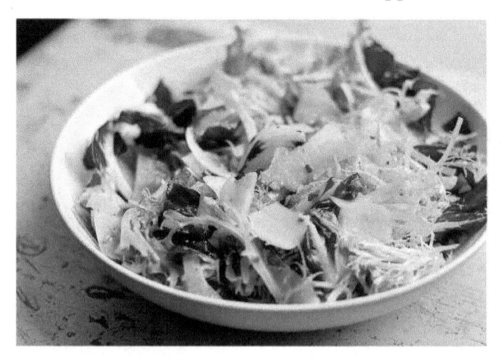

Ingredients:

- 2 heads of Radicchio, thinly sliced

- 1 head of Frisee, thinly sliced

- 2 apples, cut into very think, matchstick like slices

- 1 cup of walnuts, roasted

- 1 teaspoon balsamic vinegar

- 1 teaspoon olive oil

Preparation Time: 5 minutes

Total time: 5 minutes

Method:

- Combine the cut up radicchio, frisee, and apples in a large salad bowl, and mix well.

- Drizzle the salad with olive oil and toss. Toss walnuts over the salad, garnish with chopped mint leaves, and serve chilled.

Delicious Apple Salad (for 15 servings)

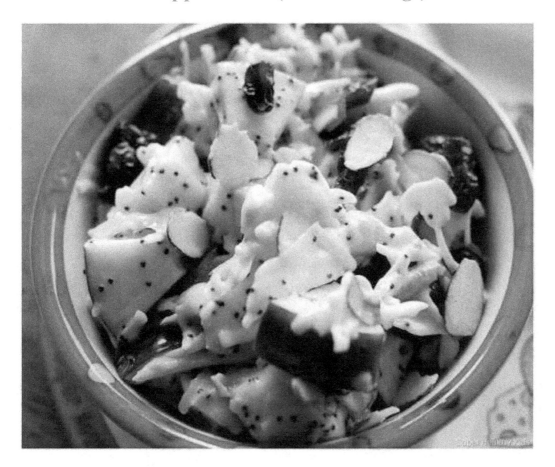

Ingredients:

- 10 Granny Smith apples, peeled, cored and chopped

- 8 ounces of canned pineapple chunks

- 1 cup pecans, chopped

- 2 cups of raisins

- 20 ounces sour cream

- 1 teaspoon granulated sugar

  Preparation Time: 10 minutes

  Total time: 10 minutes

  Method:

- In a bowl, combine the apples, raisins, chopped pecans, un-drained pineapples, and sour cream. Mix well, add the sugar and combine. Serve chilled.

Potato Salad with fresh green beans and Tarragon Dressing

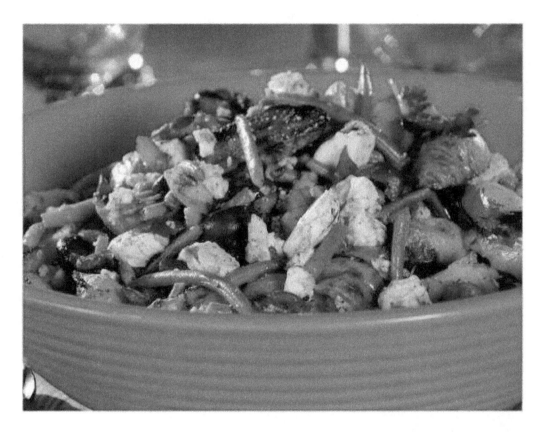

Ingredients:

- 3 pounds of potatoes

- 1 pound fresh green beans

- 1 pound bacon, lean cut with fat trimmed

- ½ cup of green onions, thinly sliced

- ¼ cup fresh parsley, finely chopped

- 1 clove garlic, minced

- 1 teaspoon dried tarragon leaves, crushed

- 1 teaspoon gluten-free dry mustard/or 1 and a ½ teaspoon ground mustard seeds

- 1 teaspoon salt

- ½ cup olive oil

- ¼ cup gluten free chicken broth

- ¼ cup tarragon vinegar

- Pepper to taste

  Preparation Time: 30 minutes

  Cooking Time: 15 minutes

  Total time: 45 minutes

  Method:

- Over medium to high heat in a non-stick pan, heat oil and fry the bacon until crisp. Drain, and crumble when cool.

- Wash the potatoes well, and slice unpeeled potatoes about ¼ inch thick. Boil in water and salt until tender and firm for around 15 minutes. Drain and cool.

- Cut the green beans into two inch pieces and steam for around 7-8 minutes, or till tender

- In a bowl, mix the light olive oil, tarragon vinegar, dried tarragon, gluten free chicken broth, minced garlic, dry mustard, salt and pepper, and whisk until well combined.

- In another bowl, mix the cooked potatoes, green beans, sliced green onions and parsley, and pour the whisked dressing over it till all vegetables are well coated. Add the crumbled bacon and mix. Serve cold.

Spinach Salad with homemade French Salad dressing (for 8 servings)

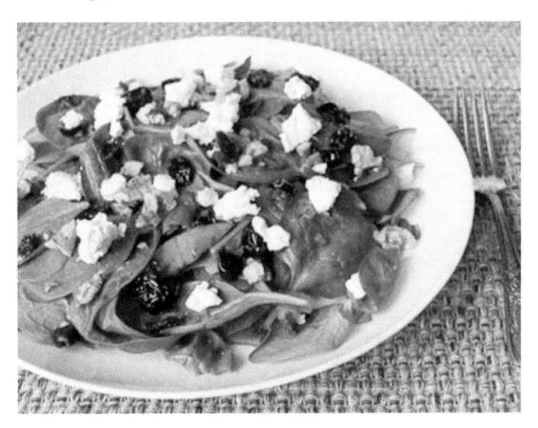

Ingredients:

• 2 pounds of spinach leaves, washed and dried

• 6 eggs, hard-boiled and finely chopped

• 8 slices bacon, lean cut and trimmed of fat, cooked and chopped

• 2 cups of red onions, thinly sliced

- 2 cups of mushrooms, thinly sliced

- ½ teaspoon of smoked paprika

  Preparation Time: 10 minutes

  Total time: 10 minutes

  Method:

- Tear the fresh spinach leaves into small pieces, and toss in the cooked and chopped gluten-free bacon pieces.

- Add the sliced onion and mushrooms, and mix well. Top the salad in a serving bowl with chopped eggs, and smoked paprika.

Bahamian Black Bean and Corn Salad (for 4 servings)

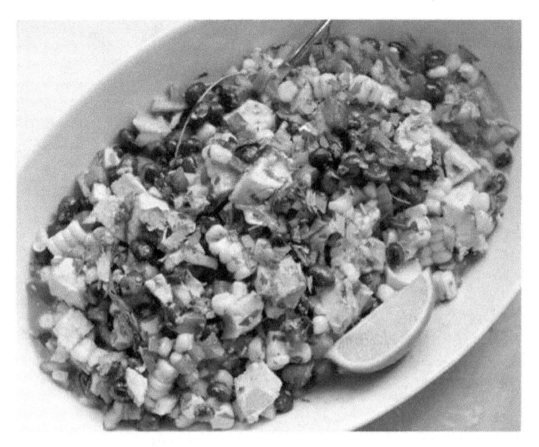

Ingredients:

- 1 can of black beans, drained

- 1 can of black-eyed peas, drained

- 1 can of corn, drained

- ½ of a large bell pepper, chopped

- ½ a large sweet onion, diced

- 2 garlic cloves, minced

- 1/3 cups of apple cider vinegar

- ¼ cup of olive oil

- 1 teaspoon sugar

- 2 tablespoons fresh cilantro, minced

- ½ teaspoon salt

- ½ a teaspoon of crushed red pepper flakes

  Preparation Time: 10 minutes

  Total time: 10 minutes

  Method:

- In a bowl, mix the beans, black-eyed peas, garlic and bell pepper.

- Place the vinegar, olive oil, sugar, salt and red pepper flakes in a bowl and whisk well.

- Pour the whisked dressing over the beans mix. Add in the minced cilantro and stir well to mix. Refrigerate and serve cold. Garnish with chopped mint leaves.

Greek Salad with Mediterranean Mint Vinaigrette (for 8 servings)

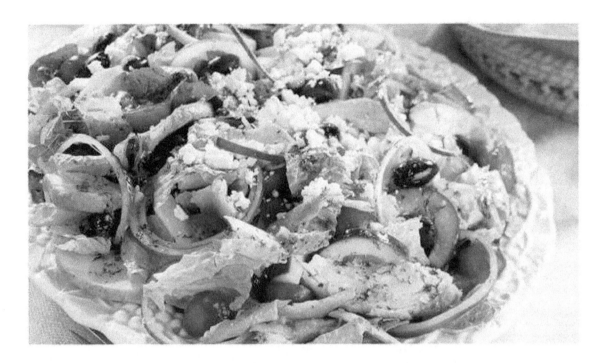

Ingredients:

- 1 head of Romaine lettuce, washed and dried

- 1 head of Bibb lettuce, washed and dried

- 3 Roma tomatoes, cut into wedges

- 1 large cucumber, thinly sliced

- 1 bell pepper, sliced into thin rings

- 1 large red onion, thinly sliced

- 1 jar un-pitted Greek Olives

- 8 ounces of Feta cheese, dry and crumbled

- ½ cup of Italian parsley, fresh, dry, and minced

- 10 Greek pepperoncini pickled peppers, from the jar

- 2 garlic cloves, minced

- 1 tablespoon of honey

- ¾ cups of olive oil

- 4 tablespoons lemon juice, freshly squeezed

- 2 teaspoons salt

- 2 teabags of "Zen" tea with lemongrass and spearmint

  <u>Preparation Time:</u> 20 minutes

  <u>Total time:</u> 20 minutes

  <u>Method:</u>

- Tear the Romaine and Bibb lettuce heads into small pieces, and arrange in rows on a platter or serving dish.

- Layer the chopped vegetables evenly over the lettuce. Top with the crumbled Feta, sliced un-pitted olives, and sliced black olives. Garnish with the minced parsley. Serve with Mediterranean Mint Vinaigrette.

- To prepare the Mediterranean Mint Vinaigrette, mix the minced garlic, salt, lemon juice, and honey in a bowl. Cut open the teabags and add the contents to the mixture. Drizzle olive oil slowly and constantly into the mixture, and whisk constantly till well mixed. Add the olive oil till you feel the dressing thicken.

- Pour the Vinaigrette over the salad, refrigerate and serve cold.

Asparagus Potato Salad (for 10 servings)

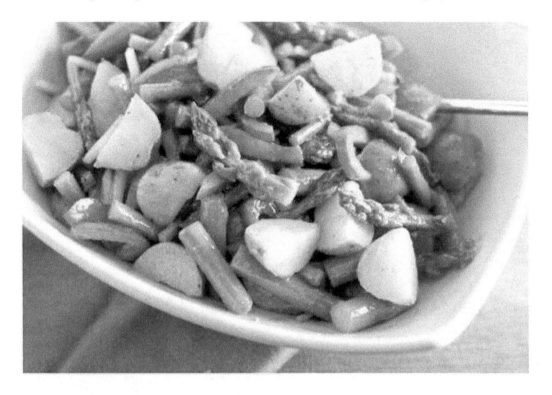

Ingredients:

• 2 pounds of potatoes, scrubbed well

• 1 cup of sweet onion, finely chopped

• 1 pound of fresh asparagus, sliced into 1 inch pieces

• 8 anchovy fillets

• 2 tablespoons lemon juice

• 1 cup of mayonnaise

• 4 teaspoons small capers, drained

• 2 tablespoons roasted red peppers, chopped

• 2 eggs, hard-boiled and cut into quarters

- 2 teaspoons yellow mustard

- 2 tablespoons sweet pickle relish

- ½ teaspoons of dried dill weed

- 1 teaspoon kosher salt

- Freshly ground black pepper

- Sweet Hungarian paprika, enough to garnish

  Preparation Time: 10 minutes

  Cooking Time: 20 minutes

  Total time: 30 minutes

  Method:

- Boil potatoes in salted water until they are tender. Drain and cool. Peel and chop into 1-inch chunks.

- Steam the asparagus until crispy and tender. Rinse in cold water and drain.

- In a bowl, combine the asparagus, potatoes, and chopped sweet onion.

- In another bowl, add the lemon juice, mayonnaise, pickle relish, dill weed, mustard, salt and pepper and whisk till well mixed and smooth. Pour this mixture over the vegetables and mix until well combined.

- Move the potato salad to a salad dish and arrange the hard-boiled egg quarters on the edge of the dish with the wedges pointing towards the outside. Arrange the anchovies in between the egg quarters.

- Sprinkle the salad with capers and roasted red peppers. Dust the salad with paprika, and chill the salad for 1 hour. Serve cold.

Wilted Spinach with Garlic (for 4 servings)

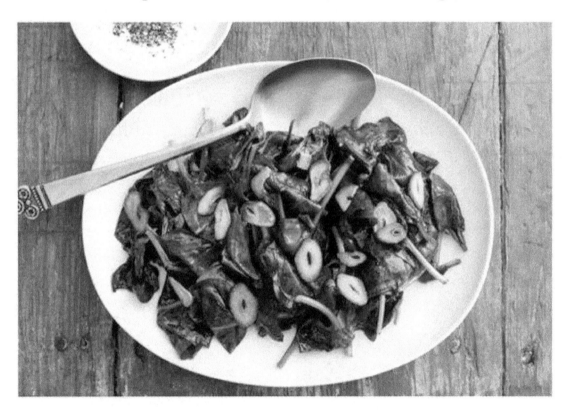

Ingredients:

- 10 ounces of baby spinach leaves

- 2 tablespoons of extra-virgin olive oil

- 4 tablespoons of parmesan cheese, crumbled

- 4 cloves of garlic, finely chopped

- 4 lemons, cut into wedges

  <u>Preparation Time:</u> 5 minutes

  <u>Cooking Time:</u> 3 minutes

  <u>Total time:</u> 8 minutes

  <u>Method:</u>

- Rinse the spinach in a colander and leave wet.

- In a large iron skillet, heat the olive oil over medium to high heat. Add the garlic and sauté until brown and giving off fragrance, for around 30 to 40 seconds.

- Add the wet spinach to the skillet and sauté until the leaves turn bright green, wilt and shrink. Cook for 2 to 3 minutes.

- Drain the oil and transfer the spinach to a servings dish. Mix in the crumbled Parmesan cheese, garnish with chopped mint leaves and lemon wedges. Serve hot or cold, as preferred.

Easy Tropical Thai Fruit Salad

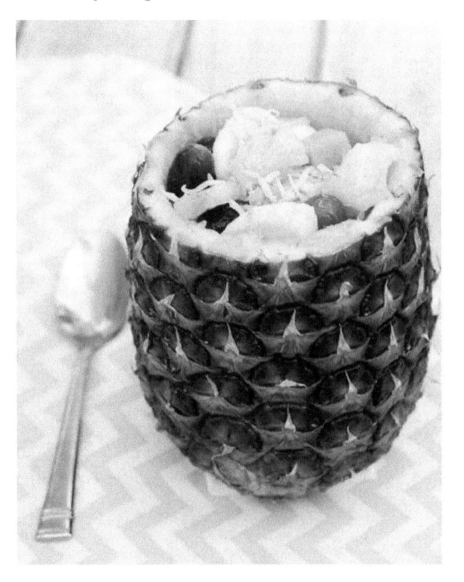

Ingredients:

- 1 whole pineapple

- 1 banana, sliced

- 1 large mango, peeled and cubed

- 1 cup of lychee fruit

- 2 cups of strawberries

- 1 star fruit, peeled and sliced (sprinkle with lemon juice to prevent browning)

- ½ cup coconut milk

- 1 tablespoon lime juice, freshly squeezed

- 2 tablespoons of castor sugar

Preparation Time: 30 minutes

Total time: 30 minutes

Method:

- Choose a fresh pineapple, and cut a thin slice off the side of the pineapple, which removes the thick needle skin and exposes the fruit inside from the side.

- Use a knife to cut around the edges inside the flesh of the fruit. Cut into cubes inside the thick skin, and using a spoon, scoop all the fleshy pineapple fruit from inside the thick skin. Save the pineapple cubes for use later.

- Mix the coconut milk, lime juice and sugar using a whisk till well mixed and all the sugar has dissolved.

- Place all the fruit inside a mixing bowl and pour the dressing over the fruit, and mix with a wooden spoon.

- Toss the salad, and scoop into the carved pineapple boat. Garnish with chopped mint leaves and serve with star fruit slices on top. Serve chilled.

CHAPTER 11: GLUTEN-FREE RECIPES FOR DESSERTS

FLOURLESS CHOCOLATE CAKE

YUMMY HOMEMADE FUDGE

CHOCOLATE MERINGUE COOKIES (FOR 3 DOZEN COOKIES)

LEMON SOUFFLÉ (FOR 8 SERVINGS)

CREAMIEST RICE PUDDING

BLUEBERRY SALAD

FLOURLESS CHOCOLATE BROWNIES (FOR 16 SERVINGS)

BAVARIAN MINTS

GLUTEN FREE FUDGE BROWNIES (FOR 16 BROWNIES)

EASY TOOTSIE ROLLS (FOR 2 DOZEN)

PECAN CLOUDS (FOR 2 DOZEN COOKIES)

APPLES BY THE FIRE (FOR 4 SERVINGS)

GLUTEN FREE RED VELVET CAKE

YUMMY PECAN PRALINES (FOR 20 PRALINES)

CHEF JOHN'S PUMPKIN CRÈME BRULEE (FOR 7 SERVINGS)

Flourless Chocolate Cake

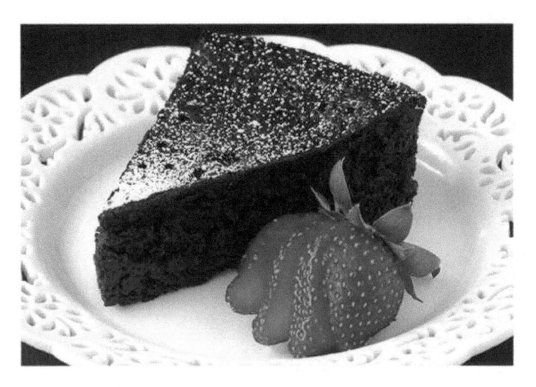

Ingredients:

- 18 squares or 1 ounce bittersweet chocolate

- 1 cup unsalted butter

- 6 eggs

- ½ cup water

- ¼ teaspoon salt

- ¾ cup white sugar

Preparation time: 15 minutes

Cooking time: 45 minutes

Method:

- Preheat oven to 300 degrees Fahrenheit or 150 degrees Celsius.

- Grease a 10-inch round cake baking pan with butter or oil and set aside.

- Combine water, salt and sugar in a small saucepan over medium heat. Stir until completely dissolved and set aside.

- Melt the bittersweet chocolate in a microwave or using a double boiler.

- Cut up the butter into smaller pieces and using an electric mixer or beater; beat the butter, one piece at a time, into the melted chocolate, till the mixture is smooth.

- Beat the sugar and water mixture, and the eggs, one at a time, into the butter and chocolate mixture.

- Pour the batter into the cake pan.

- Put the cake pan inside a larger pan, and fill the larger pan with boiling water, which reaches halfway up the cake pan.

- Put the pans into the oven, and bake for 45 minutes. It doesn't matter if the center of the cake still looks wet, that is how this cake is supposed to look.

- Chill cake overnight in the pan. To remove cake from pan, dip the bottom of the pan in hot water for a few seconds, then invert onto a platter.

Yummy Homemade Fudge

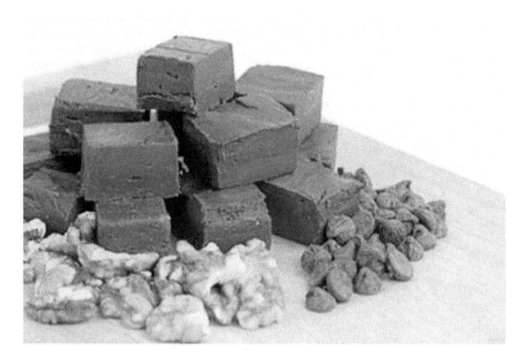

Ingredients:

- 2 ounces unsweetened chocolate, melted and cooled

- 12 ounces cream cheese, softened

- 8 cups confectioners sugar, sifted

- 1 teaspoon vanilla extract

- 2 cups walnuts, chopped

- ¼ teaspoon salt

Preparation Time: 30 minutes + 1 hour

Total time: 1 hour and 30 minutes

Method:

- Line a large square baking dish with foil.

- In a large bowl, beat the cream cheese till thick and smooth. Beat in the vanilla and salt. Then add in confectioner's sugar, adding in intervals between beatings, till mixture is smooth. Stir in the melted chocolate and walnuts.

- Pour the mixture into the baking dish and chill for an hour until it is firm. Cut into one inch squares, and serve cold with ice cream.

Chocolate Meringue Cookies (for 3 dozen cookies)

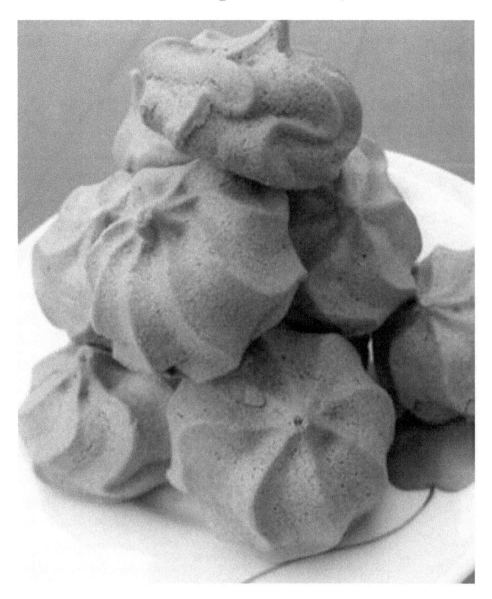

Ingredients:

- 1/3 cup semisweet chocolate chips

- 1 tablespoon unsweetened cocoa powder

- 3 egg whites

- ½ teaspoon vanilla extract

- 2/3 cup white sugar

- 1/8 teaspoon cream of tartar

  Preparation Time: 15 minutes

  Cooking Time: 30 minutes

  Total time: 45 minutes

  Method:

- Preheat oven to 300 degrees Fahrenheit or 150 degrees Celsius.

- In a bowl, beat the egg whites, vanilla, and tartar till the whites form soft peaks. Slowly add sugar while beating mixture, and beat till mixture becomes glossy and stiff peaks form. Fold in the cocoa powder and chocolate chips.

- Grease a cookie sheet. Spoon teaspoonfuls of mixture onto the tray, and bake for 25 to 30 minutes. Serve cold.

Lemon Soufflé (for 8 servings)

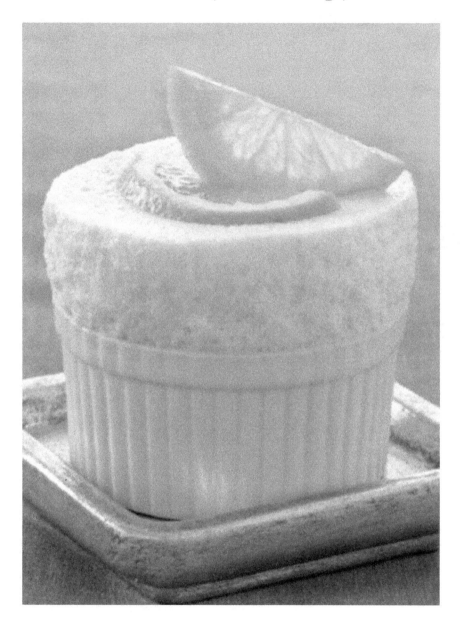

<u>Ingredients:</u>

- 2 eggs

- 3 egg yolks

- 3 egg whites

- 4 large lemons, zested and juiced

- 2 tablespoons unsalted butter, softened

- 2 teaspoons cornstarch

- ½ cup and 10 tablespoons of castor sugar

- 2 tablespoons confectioners sugar

Preparation Time: 30 minutes

Cooking Time: 15 minutes

Total time: 45 minutes

Method:

- Preheat oven to 350 degrees Fahrenheit or 175 degrees Celsius.

- Whisk eggs in a saucepan, and mix 2 lemon's zest and juice, cornstarch, and ½ cup of sugar. Cook over medium heat, stirring till mixture thickens. Then whisk for a minute on low heat. Remove from heat, and mix in the butter. Divide the mixture between 8 ramekins, each for 6 to 8 ounces.

- Whip egg whites with a mixer in a bowl till soft peaks form. Add 2 tablespoons of sugar, and resume whisking till stiff.

- Beat 8 tablespoons of sugar with egg yolks, zest and lemon juice. Fold the egg whites into the yolks, and spoon this mixture into the ramekins over the lemon curd.

- Place the ramekins on a baking sheet, and bake in oven for 15 to 17 minutes till soufflé is golden brown and risen well. Cool for 5 minutes before serving.

Creamiest Rice Pudding

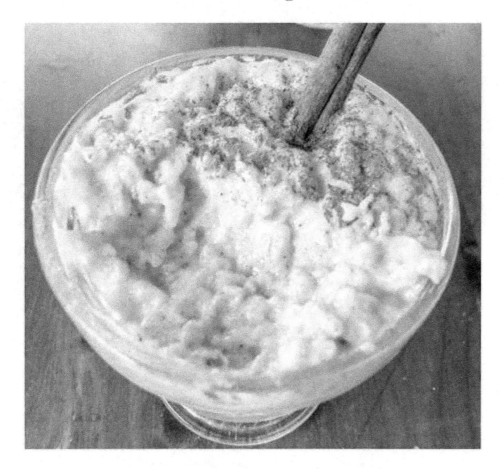

Ingredients:

- 1 cup white rice, long grain and uncooked

- ½ gallon and ¼ cup milk

- 1 cup white sugar

- 3 eggs lightly beaten

- 2 teaspoons vanilla extract

- Ground cinnamon to taste

- ¼ teaspoon salt

Preparation Time: 10 minutes + 8 hours

Cooking Time: 1 hour and 15 minutes

Total time: 8 hours

Method:

- Combine ½ gallon milk, rice and sugar in a saucepan, cover, and simmer on low heat for 1 hour, stirring at frequent intervals. After cooked, remove from heat and let rest for 10 minutes

- In a bowl, combine ¼ cup milk, vanilla and salt, and mix into the rice mixture. Cook pan on low heat for 2 minutes, stirring constantly. Pour the mixture into an 9x13 inch dish or any adequately sized dish, and cover with plastic wrap, leaving space at the corners to allow steam to escape.

- Cool pudding to room temperature, remove wrap, and garnish the pudding with ground cinnamon. Cover again with wrap and refrigerate for 8 hours at least, or overnight before serving.

Blueberry Salad

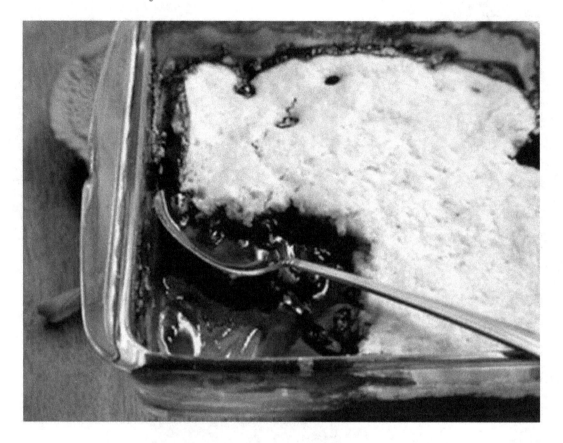

Ingredients:

- 3 ounces of packaged raspberry flavored Jell-O mix

- 2 cups of hot water

- 1 can or 20 ounces pineapple, crushed and drained

- 1 pack or 8 ounces of cream cheese

- 1 cup sour cream

- 1 teaspoon of vanilla extract

- 1 can or 21 ounces of blueberry pie filling

- ½ cup white sugar

Preparation Time: 10 minutes + 1 hour

<u>Total time:</u> 1 hour and 10 minutes

<u>Method:</u>

- Combine and mix hot water and Jell-O till dissolved. Stir in the pineapple and blueberry filling, and pour into a 9x13 or any adequately sized baking dish, and refrigerate till the mixture is firm.

- Beat together the cream cheese and sugar till smooth and creamy, then beat in vanilla and sour cream. Spread this over the gelatin mixture in the dish. Chill and serve cool.

Flourless Chocolate Brownies (for 16 servings)

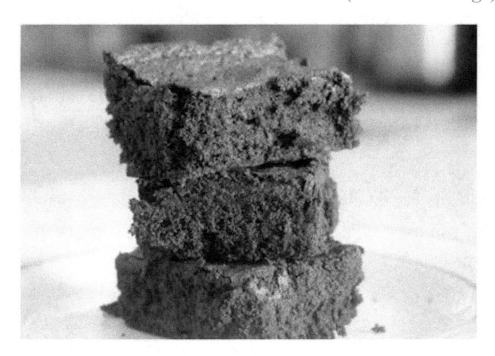

Ingredients:

- 1/3 cup brown rice flour

- ½ cup whole almonds

- 6 tablespoons unsalted butter, softened

- ½ teaspoon salt

- 2 eggs

- 1 teaspoon vanilla extract

- ½ cup bittersweet chocolate chips

- ¾ cup sugar

- 1 cup walnuts, chopped

Preparation Time: 25 minutes

Cooking Time: 25 minutes

Total time: 50 minutes

Method:

- Preheat the oven to 325 degrees Fahrenheit or 175 degrees Celsius, and place the rack in the lowest place in the oven. Line an 8x8 inch metal baking pan with baking paper.

- Add almonds to a food processer, and pulse till finely ground. Mix with rice flour.

- Set up a double boiler and add chocolate, butter and salt in the bowl over simmering water. Stir until the mixture is melted and smooth, then remove the bowl from the heat and cool for 5 minutes. Mix in the sugar, vanilla and eggs, one at a time. Fold in the flour mix and stir until well mixed. Stir in the walnuts.

- Spoon the batter into the prepared pan, spread it evenly, and bake for 20 to 25 minutes or till brownies are risen. Cool the pan on a rack, and lift out the brownies using the baking paper. Cool, cut into squares and serve with ice cream.

Bavarian Mints

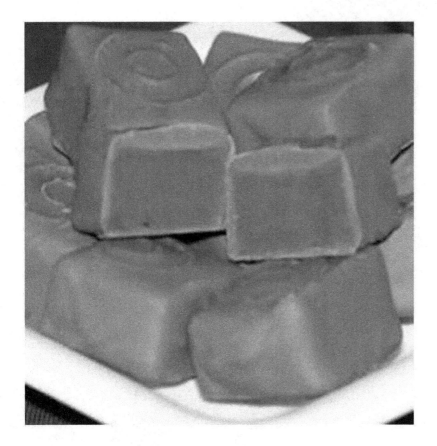

Ingredients:

- 3 cups of milk chocolate chips

- 1 ounce chopped unsweetened chocolate

- 1 can or 28 ounces sweetened condensed milk

- 1 tablespoon butter

- 1 teaspoon peppermint extract

- 1 teaspoon vanilla extract

Preparation Time: 15 minutes

Cooking Time: 25 minutes

<u>Total time:</u> 40 minutes

<u>Method:</u>

• Grease an 8x8-inch baking dish.

• Combine the chocolate chips, butter and unsweetened chocolate and heat in a saucepan over low heat, stirring constantly. Heat till melted and smooth. Remove from heat and stir in condensed milk, vanilla and peppermint extract. Mix well.

• Cool for 5 minutes, and then beat this mixture with an electric mixture for 1 minute on low speed and 1 minute on high speed. Chill the mixture for 10 minutes, beating every few minutes. Once cooled, beat with mixer again for 2 minutes. Cool for 5 minutes, then pour into the greased pan and cool. Cut into squares and serve chilled.

Gluten free Fudge Brownies (for 16 brownies)

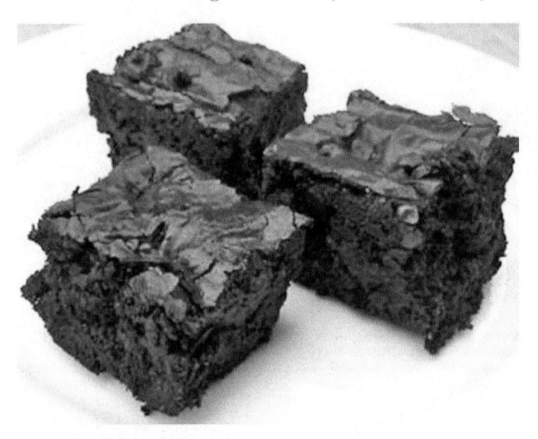

Ingredients:

- 2/3 cup gluten free baking mix

- 1 cup white sugar

- ½ cup cornstarch

- 1 teaspoon baking soda

- 2 eggs, beaten

- 1 cup brown sugar, packed

- ¾ cup unsweetened cocoa powder

- ¾ cup margarine, melted

  Preparation Time: 15 minutes

  Cooking Time: 45 minutes

  Total time: 1 hour

  Method:

- Preheat the oven to 350 degrees Fahrenheit or 175 degrees Celsius. Grease an 8x8-inch baking dish.

- Sift and mix the baking mix, white sugar, cocoa powder, cornstarch, brown sugar, and baking soda in a bowl. Pour and beat in the eggs and melted margarine, using an electric mixer for 3 to 5 minutes, till it forms a smooth batter. Spoon the mixture into the baking dish.

- Lay aluminum foil on the oven rack to prevent spills from the rising batter. Put dish on foil in the oven, bake for 40 to 45 minutes, or till a toothpick inserted into the batter comes out clean. Top with cream icing or serve with ice cream.

Easy Tootsie Rolls (for 2 dozen)

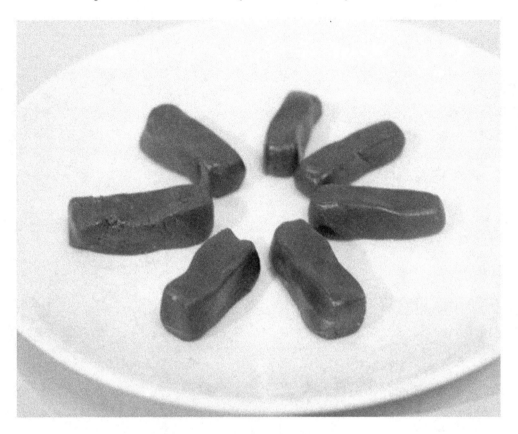

Ingredients:

- ½ cup unsweetened cocoa powder

- 3 cups confectioners sugar

- 2 tablespoons butter, cut into small chunks

- ¾ cup dry milk powder

- ½ cup white corn syrup

- 1 teaspoon vanilla extract

Preparation Time:

Total time: 15 minutes

- Mix all the ingredients together in a bowl, and knead together well till it forms a soft dough. Mold the mixture into sausage like shapes and cut into desired lengths. Serve chilled or with ice cream.

Pecan Clouds (for 2 dozen cookies)

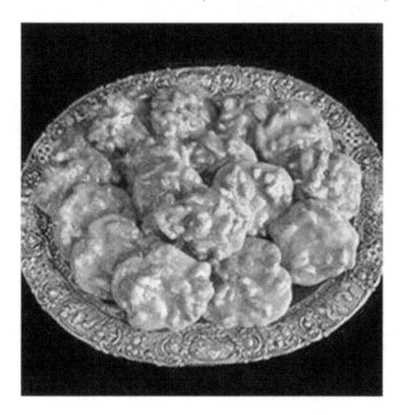

Ingredients:

- 2 cups of chopped pecans

- ¾ cup light brown sugar, packed

- 2 egg whites

- 1 teaspoon vanilla extract

Preparation Time: 15 minutes

Cooking Time: 1 hour and 30 minutes

Total time: 1 hour and 45 minutes

Method:

- Preheat the oven to 250 degrees Fahrenheit or 120 degrees Celsius. Lightly grease a cookie tray.

- In a bowl, beat egg whites using an electric mixer to form soft peaks. Add sugar in intervals during beating until the mixture forms stiff peaks.

- Stir in the vanilla extract and chopped pecans. Drop spoonfuls of mixture onto the cookie sheet. Bake in the oven for 1 hour, and then turn off heat and keep the dish in the oven for another 30 minutes, or till the cookies are dry. Serve chilled.

Apples by the fire (for 4 servings)

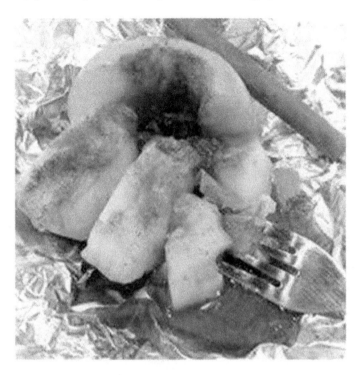

Ingredients:

- 4 Granny Smith Apples, washed and cored

- 1 teaspoon ground cinnamon

- 4 tablespoons brown sugar

  Preparation Time: 5 minutes

  Cooking Time: 10 minutes

  Total time: 15 minutes

  Method:

- Fill the empty core of each apple with 1-tablespoon brown sugar and ¼ teaspoon cinnamon.

- Wrap each apple in heavy foil, using extra foil at one end of the apple to twist into a tail.

- Light a campfire or a barbeque and place the apples in the hot coals, and let them cook for 5 to 10 minutes till they feel soft. Remove, cool for 2 minutes, then unwrap and serve hot with ice cream or whipped cream.

Gluten free Red Velvet Cake

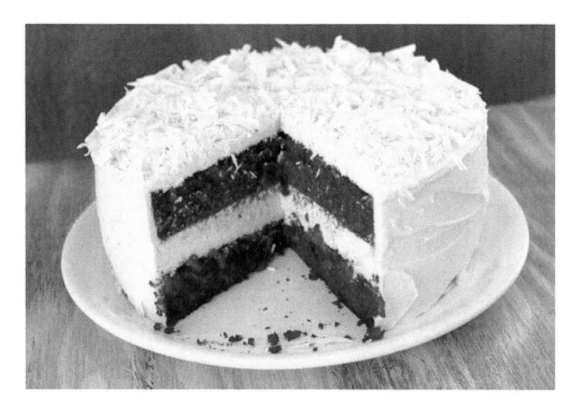

Ingredients:

- ¼ cup unsweetened cocoa powder

- ¾ cup brown rice flour

- ¾ cup sorghum flour

- ¼ cup coconut flour

- 1 and ½ cups white sugar

- 1 cup buttermilk

- ¾ cup tapioca starch

- 1 teaspoon xanthan gum

- ¼ teaspoon salt

- 1 teaspoon baking soda

- 1 cup canola oil

- 1 ounce red food coloring

- 2 eggs

- ¾ sup unsweetened applesauce

- 1 teaspoon vanilla extract

  Preparation Time: 15 minutes + 1 hour

  Cooking Time: 25 minutes

  Total time: 1 hour and 40 minutes

  Method:

- Preheat an oven to 350 degrees Fahrenheit or 175 degrees Celsius. Grease 2 round cake pans, each 9 inches, and then dust with gluten free flour.

- Whisk the three flours, baking soda, salt, xanthan gum, tapioca starch and 3 tablespoons of cocoa powder in a bowl.

- In another bowl, beat sugar and canola oil till well mixed, and then beat in eggs one at a time till fully mixed. Mix in the applesauce. Beat in the flour mixture and buttermilk alternatively in turns into the wet mixture, starting and ending with the flour mixture.

- Mix the remaining 1-tablespoon of cocoa powder with vanilla and food coloring and make a paste, which should be mixed with the batter.

- Pour the batter into the cake pans, and bake in a preheated oven for 25 minutes, or till a toothpick inserted into the cake comes out clean. Allow the cakes to cool, then remove from pan, frost between the layers and on top, and serve chilled and frosted.

Yummy Pecan Pralines (for 20 pralines)

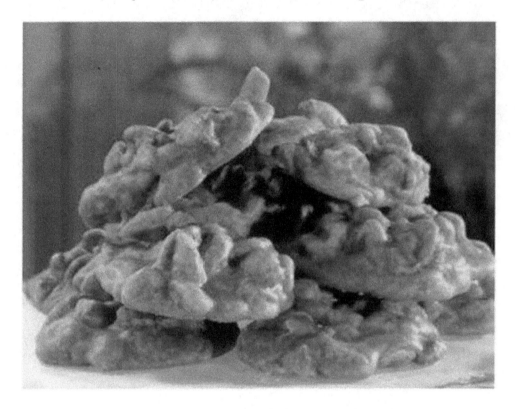

Ingredients:

- 1 cup white sugar

- 1 and ¼ cups of pecan halves

- 1 cup brown sugar

- 2 tablespoons butter

- ½ cup evaporated/condensed milk

- ¼ teaspoon vanilla extract

Preparation Time: 15 minutes + 1 hour

Cooking Time: 15 minutes

<u>Total time:</u> 1 hour and 30 minutes

<u>Method:</u>

- Grease a baking tray with oil or butter.

- Mix the brown and white sugar and milk in a saucepan over medium heat. Mix in the vanilla, pecans and butter and heat without stirring. Heat till a small amount of this mixture forms a soft ball when dropped into cold water, and can be flattened when removed from the water. When this happens, remove from heat and cool for 5 minutes.

- Beat this mixture till it is thick, then pour onto the baking try and let it rest until it is firm. Cut into squares and serve chilled.

Chef John's Pumpkin Crème Brulee (for 7 servings)

Ingredients:

* 1 cup pumpkin puree

* 3 egg yolks

* 1 cup heavy cream

* ½ cup white sugar

* ½ cup brown sugar

* ¼ teaspoon ground cinnamon

* ¼ teaspoon ground nutmeg

* ½ teaspoon ground allspice

* 1 pinch of salt

  Preparation Time: 10 minutes + 2 hours

  Cooking Time: 35 minutes

  Total time: 2 hours and 45 minutes

  Method:

* Preheat the oven to 325 degrees Fahrenheit or 165 degrees Celsius.

* In a large bowl, whisk the egg yolks and brown sugar, and then stir in the puree, allspice, cream, cinnamon, nutmeg and salt. Divide the mixture between 7 5-inch ramekins, about ½ an inch from the top.

- Half fill a deep baking dish with hot water and place the ramekins in the dish so that water reaches halfway up their sides.

- Bake in the oven for 30 to 35 minutes or till the mixture in the ramekins is set. Remove from oven and refrigerate for 2 hours or until fully chilled.

- Sprinkle a tablespoon of sugar over each cream Brulee. Use a chefs torch to melt the sugar on top for 1 to 2 minutes or until it is dark brown and crispy. Cool before serving.

CHAPTER 12: GLUTEN-FREE RECIPES FOR KIDS ON GLUTEN FREE DIETS

Gluten free Chocolate Chip Cookies (for 3 dozen cookies)

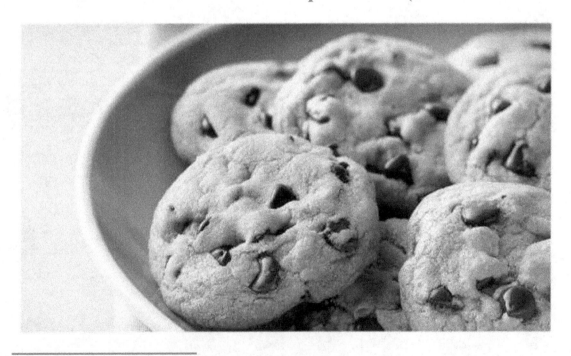

- ¾ cup softened butter

- ¼ cup white sugar

- 1 and ¼ cups packed brown sugar

- 1 teaspoon baking soda

- ¼ cup egg substitute

- 1 teaspoon salt

- 1 teaspoon baking powder

- 1 teaspoon gluten free vanilla extract

- 12 ounces semisweet chocolate chips

Preparation Time: 15 minutes

Cooking time: 10 minutes

Total time: 25 minutes

Method:

- Preheat oven to 375 degrees Fahrenheit or 190 degrees Celsius. Grease a baking tray or line a tray with a baking sheet.

- In a bowl, beat butter and sugar together till light and creamy.

- Gradually beat in vanilla extract and egg substitute till you have a smooth mixture.

- Sift gluten-free flour mix, baking powder, baking soda, and salt. Fold in the sifted mixture to the butter mixture until smooth and well blended. Last, stir in the chocolate chips.

- Using a spoon, drop cookie dough, and press the top flat with the back of the spoon, onto the baking pan or baking sheet, 2 inches apart.

- Bake in a preheated oven for 8 to 10 minutes until golden brown. Cool the cookies on a baking sheet for 2 minutes and then cool on a wire rack. Serve hot with ice cream or serve cool, as preferred.

Gluten Free Cheese and Herb Pizza Crust (Makes 1 pizza crust. This recipe does not include toppings; you can top the crust in any way that you want.)

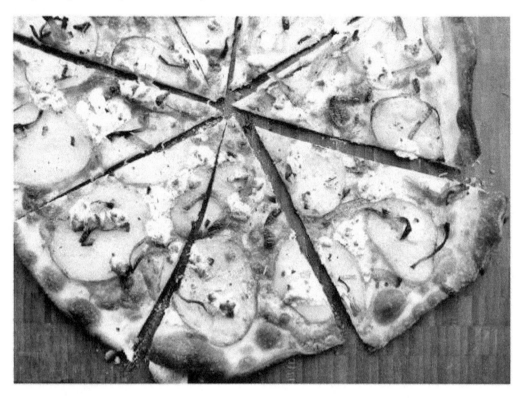

Ingredients:

- ¾ cup gluten free all purpose baking flour

- ¼ cup garbanzo bean flour

- ¼ cup tapioca starch

- 1 and ½ teaspoons baking powder

- ¼ cup cornstarch

- ¼ cup grated Parmesan cheese

- 1 teaspoon xanthan gum

- 1 teaspoon dried oregano

- 1 teaspoon Italian seasoning

- ½ teaspoon salt

- 1 egg

- 2 teaspoon white sugar

- ½ teaspoon minced garlic

- 1 cup lukewarm water

- 1 and a ½ teaspoons olive oil

- ½ teaspoon apple cider vinegar

- 1 package (1/4 ounce) package active dry yeast

  Preparation Time: 15 minutes

  Cooking Time: 30 minutes

  Total Time: 45 minutes

<u>Method:</u>

- Preheat oven to 425 degrees Fahrenheit or 220 degrees Celsius. Grease a 15-inch pizza pan with oil, butter or cooking spray.

- Mix all purpose baking flour, garbanzo bean flour, cornstarch, baking powder, tapioca starch, xanthan gum, Parmesan cheese, oregano, salt, and Italian seasoning in a bowl and set aside.

- Dissolve 1 teaspoon white sugar in lukewarm water in a small bowl. Sprinkle the yeast over the water, and set aside in a dry, warm place for 3 to 5 minutes till the mixture is foamy.

- Add the egg, olive oil, sugar, garlic, and vinegar in a bowl and beat until the mixture is smooth.

- Add the yeast mixture to the egg mixture, whisk in, and stir in flour mixture till it is smooth and no dry lumps remain.

- Mix the mixture well into dough, roll it, and press it into the prepared pizza pan. Make sure the outer edge is thicker than the center of the dough.

- Cook the crust in the preheated oven for 10 to 12 minutes, till the dough rises and is slightly firm.

- Top the crust with your desirable toppings, and continue baking at the same temperature till cheese on top has melted and set, and the crust is golden brown. Bake for around 20 to 30 minutes.

- Remove the pizza from the pan and cool on the oven rack for 5 minutes to allow the crust to crisp. This step is optional if crispier crusts are preferred. Otherwise, remove from pan and serve immediately.

Gluten Free Banana Bread (for 8 servings)

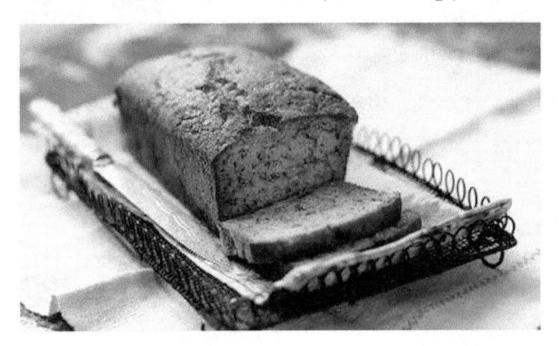

Ingredients:

- 1 cup of gluten free all purpose baking flour

- ½ a teaspoon of baking powder

- 1 egg, lightly beaten

- 3 ripe and sweet bananas, mashed with a fork

- 1 and a ½ tablespoons of maple syrup

- ¼ teaspoon of salt

- ¼ cup butter

- ¼ cup turbinado sugar

  <u>Preparation time:</u> 15 minutes

  <u>Cooking time:</u> 30 minutes

  <u>Total time:</u> 45 minutes

  <u>Method:</u>

- Preheat an oven to 350 degrees Fahrenheit or 175 degrees Celsius. Also grease a loaf pan, preferably 9x5 inches, with butter, oil or cooking spray.

- Combine the flour, baking powder and salt in a large bowl. In another bowl, using an electric mixer or beater, cream the butter and sugar well. Add the maple syrup, eggs and mashed bananas into the butter and sugar and blend well, till well light and fluffy. Add the banana mixture to the flour mixture and mix well until the batter is soft and moist.

- Pour the batter into the greased loaf pan. Bake in the preheated oven for 20 to 30 minutes till the batter has risen. Use a toothpick or fork to check whether the loaf is done; if the toothpick or fork is inserted into the center of the batter and come out clean, the loaf is cooked. For people using other trays, such as muffin or cupcake trays, bake for around 15 minutes or until a fork or toothpick comes out clean when inserted into the center of the muffin. Serve hot, warm or cold with margarine, honey or jam of your choice.

Brown Rice, Broccoli, Cheese and Walnut Surprise (for 8 servings)

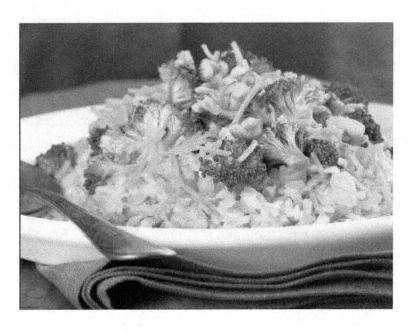

Ingredients:

- 1 cup walnuts, chopped

- 2 pound fresh broccoli florets

- 2 cups cheddar cheese, shredded

- 2 onions, chopped

- 2 tablespoons butter

- 2 cups uncooked brown rice

- 2 cups vegetable broth

- 1 teaspoon garlic, minced

- ¼ teaspoon ground black pepper

- 1 teaspoon salt

Preparation Time: 15 minutes

Cooking Time: 25 minutes

Total time: 40 minutes

Method:

- Preheat the oven to 350 degrees Fahrenheit or 175 degrees Celsius.

- Toast the walnuts on a small baking tray in the oven for 6 to 8 minutes till they are crispy, brown and well toasted.

- In a saucepan, melt the butter over medium heat. Add the garlic and onions, and cook for 3 minutes, stirring occasionally. Stir in the rice and broth, and bring the mixture to a boil. Then cover and simmer on low heat for 8 to 10 minutes till the liquid is absorbed.

- In a casserole dish, place the broccoli and season with pepper and salt. Cover, and microwave till the broccoli is tender.

- In a serving dish, move and arrange the rice and add the broccoli on top. Garnish with walnuts and cheese, and serve warm.

Pan Seared Salmon (for 6 servings)

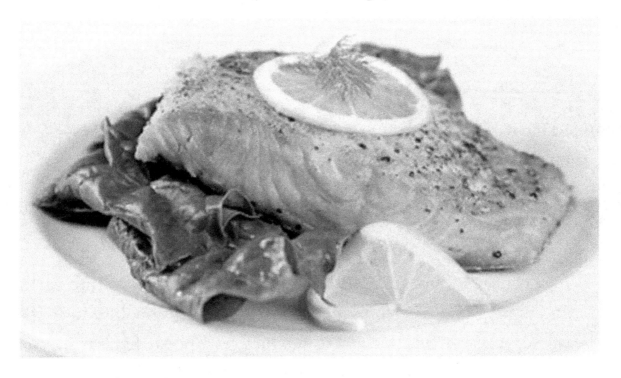

Ingredients:

- 6 salmon fillets, each of 6 ounces

- ½ tablespoons olive oil

- 6 lemon slices

- 3 tablespoons of capers

- ¼ teaspoon salt

- ¼ teaspoon pepper

Preparation Time: 10 minutes

Cooking Time: 10 minutes

Total time: 20 minutes

Method:

- Heat a pan or iron skillet over medium heat for a few minutes.

- Cover the salmon with olive oil, and cook in the pan for 3 minutes on high heat. Sprinkle with salt, pepper and capers. Turn the salmon, and cook for another 5 minutes till browned. Cook till the salmon is tender and flakes easily with a fork.

- Transfer the salmon to individual plates, garnish with lemon slices, and serve hot. Serve with tartar sauce, yoghurt mint sauce, boiled vegetables, or on a bed of pasta or boiled rice.

Spicy Burgers (for 4 servings)

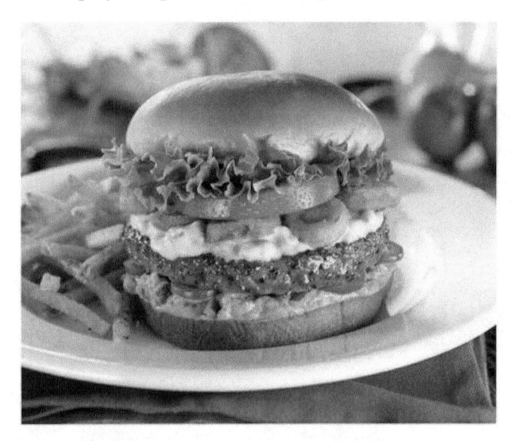

Ingredients:

- 1 pound of ground beef

- 1 jalapeno pepper, seeded and minced

- 1 teaspoon garlic, minced

- 1 tablespoon fresh cilantro, chopped

- ½ teaspoon crushed red pepper flakes

- ½ poblano chile pepper, seeded and minced

- ½ habanero pepper, seeded and minced

- ½ teaspoon ground cumin

Preparation Time: 15 minutes

Cooking Time: 10 minutes

Total time: 25 minutes

Method:

- Preheat the grill on high heat.

- In a large bowl, mix together all the ingredients with a metal spoon or your hands. Using wet hands, mold handfuls of the mixture into burger patties.

- Grease the grill with butter or oil and cook the burgers for 5 minutes on each side till soft, brown and well done. Serve inside a bun with potato fries.

Gluten free Chicken Nuggets (for 4 servings)

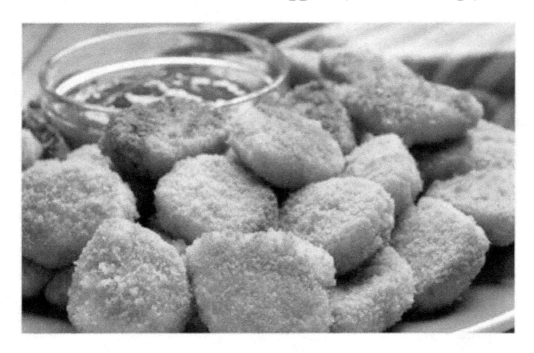

Ingredients:

- 4 chicken breast halves, boneless and skinless, chopped into small pieces

- 2 eggs

- 1 cups of corn square cereal

- 1/3 cup rice flour

- ¼ cup oil for frying

Preparation Time: 15 minutes

Cooking Time: 5 minutes

Total time: 20 minutes

Method:

- Blend cereal in a food processor till it looks like breadcrumbs, and then move to a bowl.

- Add the oil to a skillet and heat over medium to high heat.

- Beat two eggs in one bowl, and spread the rice flour on one plate. Cover the chicken pieces in rice flour, and then dip in beaten egg and then coat in the cereal. Repeat for all chicken, and put on another plate.

- Fry the chicken nuggets in hot oil until browned and cooked through, for 3 minutes on each side. Serve with fries.

Easy Gluten-free Macaroni and Cheese (for 4 servings)

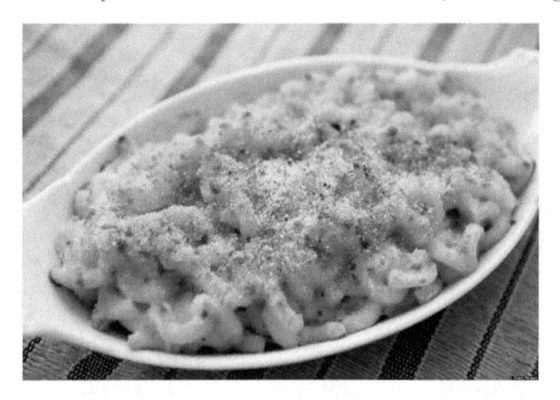

Ingredients:

- 5 ounces of gluten free elbow pasta

- 3 tablespoons of butter

- 2 cups milk

- 2 and a ½ tablespoons cornstarch

- ¾ teaspoons salt

- 2 cups cheddar cheese, shredded

- ¼ teaspoon mustard powder

- ¼ teaspoon paprika

- ½ teaspoon softened butter

- 1 gluten free bread slice, toasted and crumbed

  Preparation Time: 15 minutes

  Cooking Time: 45 minutes

  Total time: 1 hour

  Method:

- Preheat oven to 375 degrees Fahrenheit or 190 degrees Celsius. Grease an 8x8-inch baking dish with butter or oil.

- Boil a large pot of lightly salted water, add macaroni, and cook for 8 minutes, or till tender but firm, stirring occasionally. Drain, and cool under running cold water.

- Place 2 and a ½ tablespoons of butter, mustard powder and salt in a saucepan over medium heat. Cook till well mixed and heated, and remove from heat.

- Whisk cornstarch and milk in a bowl to smooth consistency, and then add in the mustard and butter mixture. Combine well, return the saucepan to medium heat, and cook the mixture, stirring constantly, for 4 to 6 minutes, or until the sauce is smooth and thick. Remove from heat.

- Add 1 and 1/3 cups of cheddar cheese to the sauce, and allow it to melt. Add the pasta into the cheese sauce and mix well, then pour this into the greased baking dish. Top the mixture with the remaining cheddar cheese, paprika, breadcrumbs and ½ tablespoon of butter. Bake in the oven for 30 minutes or till the cheese on top has melted and the top is golden brown and crunchy.

CHAPTER 13: GLUTEN-FREE SLOW COOKER RECIPES

Baked Slow Cooker Chicken (for 6 servings)

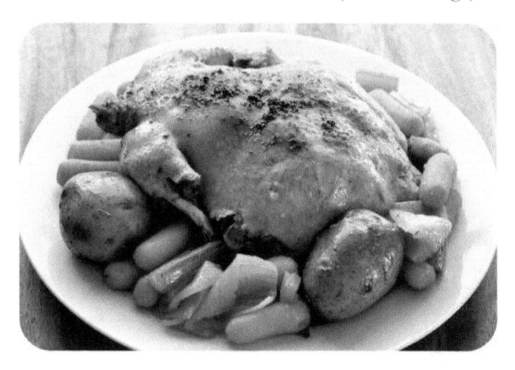

Ingredients:

- 1 whole chicken, or a 3 pound chicken

- 1 teaspoon paprika

- Salt and pepper to taste

  Preparation time: 20 minutes

  Cooking time: 10 hours

  Total time: 10 hours and 20 minutes

  Method:

- Scrunch a few pieces of aluminum foil into 3-4 inch balls, and place them at the bottom of the slow cooker you are going to use.

- Rinse the chicken well, outside and inside the chicken cavity, using cold running water. Pat dry, and season the chicken well with salt, pepper and paprika. Place the chicken in the slow cooker above the crumpled aluminum foil.

- Set the slow cooker to "High" for 1 hour, and cook. After 1 hour, turn the cooker to "Low" for around 8 to 10 hours, or till the chicken is no longer pink and the juices run clear.

Barbecued Beef (for 12 servings)

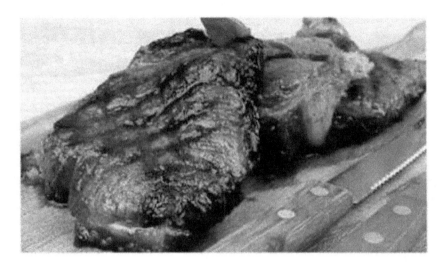

Ingredients:

- 1 boneless chuck roast, or a 4 pound boneless chuck roast

- 2 tablespoons Worcestershire sauce

- 1 and a ½ cups ketchup

- ¼ cup red wine vinegar

- ¼ cup packed brown sugar

- 1 teaspoon liquid smoke flavoring

- 2 tablespoons prepared Dijon-style mustard

- ½ teaspoon salt

- ¼ teaspoon ground black pepper

- ¼ teaspoon garlic powder

Preparation time: 20 minutes

Cooking time: 10 hours

<u>Total time:</u> 10 hours and 20 minutes

<u>Method:</u>

- Combine ketchup, liquid smoke flavoring, brown sugar, Worcestershire sauce, red wine vinegar and Dijon-style mustard in a bowl. Add salt, pepper and garlic powder and mix well.

- Place chuck roast in a slow cooker. Pour the ketchup mixture over the chuck roast, cover, and cook on "Low" in the slow cooker for 8

  to 10 hours.

- Remove the chuck roast from the slow cooker, shred with a fork to break the meat down into flakes. Put meat back into the cooker and mix well with the sauce till all meat is coated evenly. Continue to cook for another hour. Serve with mint garnishing.

Charley's Slow Cooker Mexican Style Meat (for 12 servings)

Note: Beef, Chicken, Pork, or Venison can be used. See the end of the recipe for variations.

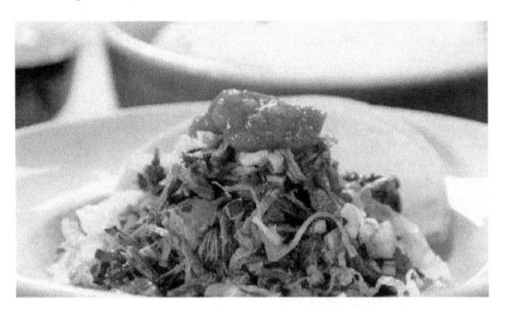

Ingredients:

- 1 chuck roast (4 pounds)

- 2 tablespoons olive oil

- 1 large onion, chopped

- 5 ounces of hot pepper sauce

- 1 teaspoon salt

- 1 teaspoon garlic powder

- 1 teaspoon ground black pepper

- 1 and ¼ cups of diced green chili pepper

- 1 teaspoon of chili powder

- 1 teaspoon ground cayenne pepper

  <u>Preparation Time:</u> 30 minutes + 20 minutes

  <u>Cooking Time:</u> 8 hours

  <u>Total time:</u> 8 hours and 50 minutes

  <u>Method:</u>

- Trim the meat of any excess fat, and season well with salt and pepper. In a large iron skillet, heat olive oil over medium to high heat. Cook and brown the beef on all sides.

- In a slow cooker, add the meat and the chopped onions. Season with the chili powder, chili peppers, cayenne pepper, garlic powder and hot pepper sauce, and mix well. Add water over the beef, covering 1/3 of the meat.

- Cover the cooker, and cook on High heat for 6 hours, checking periodically to ensure there is adequate liquid at the bottom of the cooker.

- Change the cooker heat to low, and cook another 3 to 4 hours, or until the meat is tender and falls apart easily when tested with a fork.

- In a bowl, add the roast from the cooker and shred it using a fork. Serve as desired, in sandwiches, tacos, spaghetti, burritos, or as desired.

- For pork, chicken and venison, remove the skin before cooking and reduce the cooking time to 4 hours on High heat or alternatively, 8 hours on Low heat.

Beckey's Slow Cooker Gluten-free Thai Chicken Curry (for 8 servings)

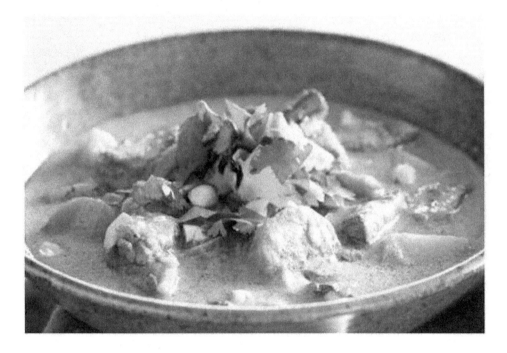

Ingredients:

- 8 chicken thighs

- ½ cup sugar snap peas

- 2 cans or 28 ounces of coconut milk

- 4 tablespoons of peanut butter

- 2 teaspoons red curry powder

- 4 tablespoons liquid amino acid

- 1 sweet onion, chopped

- 1 teaspoon brown sugar

- 2 teaspoons of red curry paste

- 1 red bell pepper, chopped

- ½ cup fresh cilantro, chopped

- 2 teaspoons dried basil

Preparation Time: 15 minutes

Cooking Time: 3 hours and 10 minutes

Total time: 3 hours and 25 minutes

Method:

- Add all ingredients together in a slow cooker except the chicken and snap peas, starting with the liquids, then the powders and then the remaining ingredients. Stir well, and then place the chicken thighs in the cooker.

- Cook on High heat for 3 hours, till the chicken is cooked and not raw and pink in the center. Add the snap peas now, stir, and cook for another 10 minutes till peas are heated through. Serve hot.

Slow Cooker Tapioca Pudding (for 8 servings)

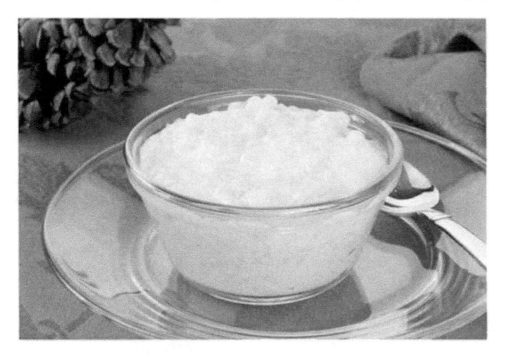

Ingredients:

1. 4 cups of milk

• 2 eggs, beaten

• ½ cup of small pearl tapioca

• 2/3 cup white sugar

Preparation Time: 5 minutes

Cooking Time: 3 hours

Total time: 3 hours and 5 minutes

Method:

• Stir together all the ingredients in a slow cooker, and mix well. Cover, and cook on Medium heat for 3 hours or for 6 hours on Low heat, stirring every half an hour. Serve warm.

CHAPTER 14: GLUTEN-FREE RECIPES FOR HEALTHY, TASTY SMOOTHIES

Choco-peanut-banana Smoothie (for 2 servings)

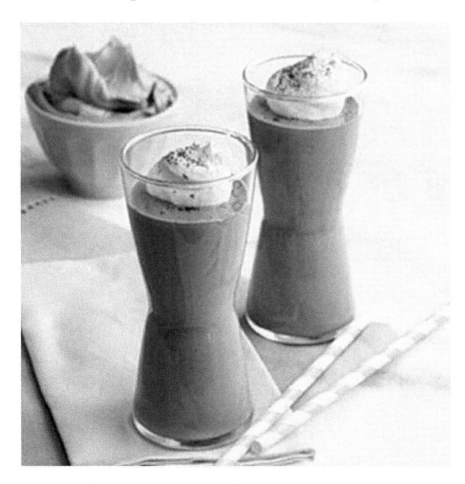

Ingredients:

- 2 bananas, thinly sliced

- 1 cup milk, skimmed

- 4 tablespoons chocolate syrup

- 4 tablespoons peanut butter

Preparation Time: 5 minutes

Total time: 5 minutes

Method:

- Blend all the ingredients together in a blender at high speed till thick and smooth. Serve cold.

California Smoothie (for 2 servings)

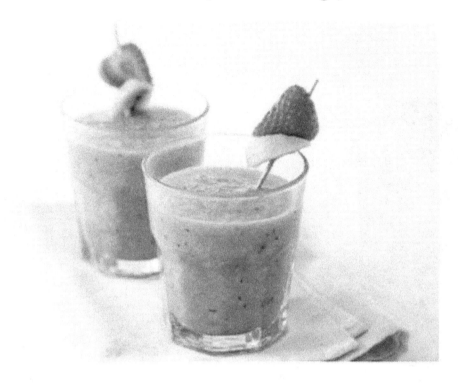

Ingredients:

- 15 large frozen strawberries

- 2/3 cup of orange juice

- 2 packs or 16 ounces of lemon yoghurt

- 1 cup ice, crushed

Preparation Time: 10 minutes

Total time: 10 minutes

Method:

- Blend all ingredients together in blender at full speed till thick and smooth. Serve cold.

Vodka Smoothie (for 4 servings)

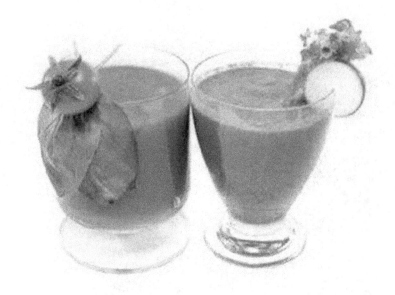

Ingredients:

- 6 ounces of vodka

- 1 cup frozen strawberries

- 18 ounces or orange juice

- 4 scoops orange sherbet

- 1 cup ice, crushed

Preparation Time: 10 minutes

Total time: 10 minutes

Method:

- In a blender, blend all ingredients at high speed till thick and smooth. Serve chilled.

Blueberry Smoothie (for 2 servings)

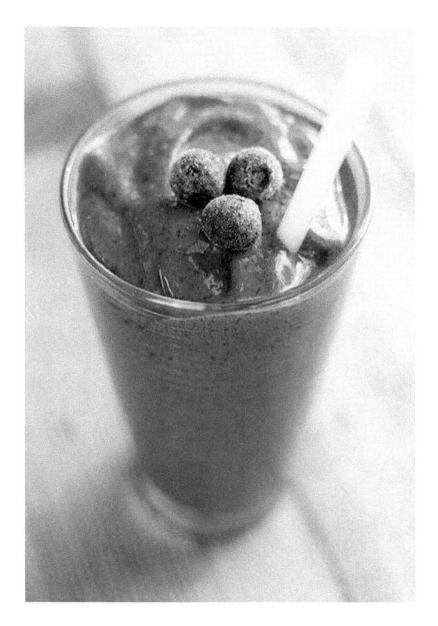

Ingredients:

- 1 and ¼ cups of Blueberry Juice Cocktail, chilled

- 1 cup vanilla yoghurt or frozen yoghurt

- ¾ cup of fresh Blueberries, washed well

Preparation Time: 5 minutes

Total time: 5 minutes

<u>Method:</u>

- Blend the blueberries and blueberry juice cocktail in a blender at high speed till smooth. Add yoghurt, blend again till thick and well combined. Serve chilled.

Mocha Smoothie (for 2 servings)

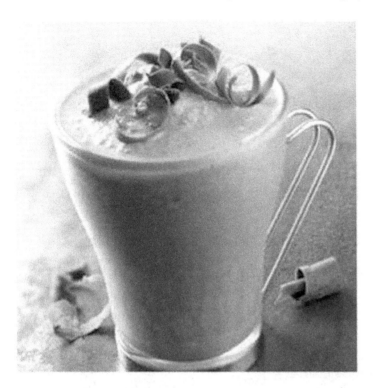

Ingredients:

- 2 tablespoons hot chocolate mix

- 2 cups ice, crushed

- ½ cup brewed coffee

- 1 and a ½ cup coconut milk

- 6 tablespoons of turbinado sugar

- 2 tablespoons vanilla extract

Preparation Time: 10 minutes

Total time: 10 minutes

Method:

- In a blender, blend together all the aforementioned ingredients till smooth. Serve chilled.

APPENDIX

In the beginning, it's a little harder to streamline your diet because of confusion over what food is gluten-free and what isn't. The most important thing is to get your basics right. Once you learn the foundation of what should be excluded and what is good for the diet, in time, keeping up with it will become easier.

The most common gluten free grain products that should be part of your diet include:

- Amaranth

- Corn flour

- Millet

- Quinoa

- Buckwheat

- Sorghum

- Cornmeal

- Vegetable Oils

- Montina

- Rice (brown, basmati, white and enriched)

- Grits

- Soy

Common staple foods that are safe to be a part of your gluten-free diet include:

- Beans

- Butter

- Legumes

- Cheese (most types, but be careful to read labels)

- Lean meats

- Margarine

- Milk

- Fresh Fruits

- Fresh Vegetables

- Yoghurt (Plan yoghurt is acceptable, flavored yoghurt requires label checks)

- Fresh seafood (read labels for frozen seafood)

The following products are also gluten-free, when and if needed to be used in recipes:

- Glucose syrup

- Lactose

- Starch

- Sucrose

- Vinegar (except Malt Vinegar)

- Dextrose

- Annatto

- Silicon Dioxide

- Oat gum

- Lecithin

- Malodextrin (it can even be consumed when it is made from wheat)

You can also seek help from online sources that give guidance on gluten-free diets, and help with finding gluten free recipes, restaurants, and buying gluten free products, etc. The following websites can be accessed using the links below:

- Glutenfree.com (https://www.glutenfree.com/#filters/)

- Blog on eating gluten free (http://glutenfreegoddess.blogspot.com/)

- Gluten Free Cooking School (http://www.glutenfreecookingschool.com/)

- Purchasing Gluten free products (http://www.glutenfreepalace.com/)

- Gluten Free Living (http://www.glutenfreeliving.com/)

- Gluten free Girl and the Chef (http://glutenfreegirl.com/)

- Everything about being Gluten Free (https://simplygluten-free.com/)

- Gluten free Doctor (http://glutenfreedoctor.com/)

- Cooking on the Weekends (http://cookingontheweekends.com/category/gluten-free/)

- Gluten free Mall (https://www.glutenfreemall.com/catalog/)

- Gluten free Foods (http://www.glutenfree-foods.co.uk/)

- Gluten Free on a Shoestring (http://glutenfreeonashoestring.com/)

- Delight Gluten free Magazine (http://www.delightglutenfree.com/)

- Genius Gluten Free (http://www.geniusglutenfree.com/en_GB/?site=geniusfoods&clear=true)

- Glutino (http://www.glutino.com/)

- Too Good to be Gluten Free (http://toogoodtobeglutenfree.com/)

- Gluten Free life (http://gfreelife.com/)

CONCLUSION

Correct diet is the foundation of good health, which is why nutritious eating is so important for your body to feel good and to look good. We hoped that you liked these recipes

Finally, if you enjoyed this book, then I'd like to ask you for a favor, would you be kind enough to leave a review for this book on Amazon? It'd be greatly appreciated!

Click here to leave a review for this book on Amazon!

Thank you and good luck!

CPSIA information can be obtained
at www.ICGtesting.com
Printed in the USA
BVHW061401230621
610214BV00004B/451